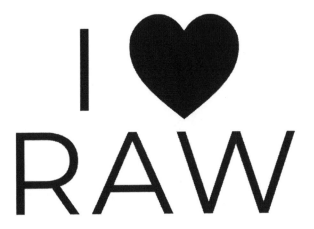

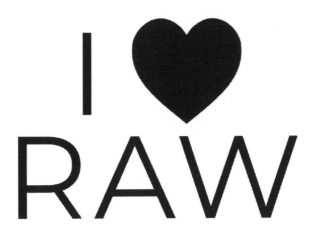

I ♥ RAW

A How-To Guide for
Reconnecting to Yourself and the Earth
through Plant-Based Living

CHRISTY HARDEN, M.S., M.A.

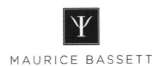

MAURICE BASSETT

I ♥ Raw: A How-To Guide for Reconnecting to Yourself and the Earth through Plant-Based Living

Maurice Bassett
P.O. Box 839
Anna Maria, FL 34216

Contact the publisher:
MauriceBassett@gmail.com
www.MauriceBassett.com

Editor: Chris Nelson
Cover design: David Michael Moore
Cover photograph: Rudy Meyers

ISBN: 978-1-60025-091-0

Library of Congress Control Number: 2020934386

First Edition

To the animals

Acknowledgments

A partial list:

- ♥ **Maurice Bassett**. For believing in me and my visions and helping to facilitate their birth into the world.
- ♥ **Chris Nelson**. Your patience, kindness and editing are all magic; you've become a real friend.
- ♥ **Kevin Benevedo**. Thank you for your friendship, your authenticity, your humor, your eagle-eye editing and persistent belief in me and my expression. I so appreciate your willingness to be on this journey with me.
- ♥ **Kyle Cease**. What a ride, babe. You inspire me and not only support but demand the freedom of my heart; what a gift. Through it all, you remind me of who I am when I forget: just this moment. It's been and continues to be an absolute honor.
- ♥ **Dylan and Marissa Predko**. Thank you for your love and support. I love you and Phoebe so much.
- ♥ **My parents**. Forever gratitude for raising me to value and enjoy health, nature, writing and books.
- ♥ And **Vivien**. I'm in heaven and cherish every moment of getting to know you better and better every moment. You are a delight. I love you and your big joyful, animal-loving heart with all of mine, Teeny.
    - ♥ In memory of my dad.

Contents

You must live life in its very elementary forms. The Mexicans have a very nice word for it: *Pura vida*. It doesn't mean just purity of life, but the raw, stark-naked quality of life.

~ Werner Herzog

Foreword

I don't know anyone who lives what they teach more than Christy. She lives and loves raw food. I've tried so many times to just get her to take a bite out of one thing that's been cooked, and she'll usually just kind of look at it like a squirrel debating whether or not to eat a Snickers bar—and pass.

I've seen her live a miraculously healthy life. I've watched her reverse her aging—every year she seems a year younger. And because of this woman I've also discovered how much I appreciate my own health, animals, trees, nature and the world. She taught me how to love a tree, which is really my way of saying that she teaches us how to appreciate everything that gives us love without asking for anything in return. She's a warrior for the unheard. She's here to reconnect us with a world that is trying to nurture us, heal us and bring joy into our lives. Christy is on a mission to make sure we all know we can live much more vibrant, magical, synchronistic and healthy lives—and that we don't have to suffer nearly as much as we do.

This whole book is inspired, but even just the little shifts you'll get by reading it can change the entire course of your life and help you create a more vibrant connection to yourself, your family and the world. Not to mention a healthier life and greater longevity.

That's why NOT reading this book might be the biggest

mistake you never knew you made. Do not pass it up! Christy is a brilliant, beautiful and powerful woman, and now more than ever the world needs her *and* her vision of who we truly are.

Kyle Cease
Los Angeles, CA
May, 2020

Preface: My Journey

My journey from the Standard American Diet (SAD) to the raw vegan lifestyle—and to true health—happened in fits and starts.

Even as a full-term infant born to generally healthy parents, I began life on shaky ground. As a child I suffered from severe food sensitivities/intolerances and asthma, and I was often ill with pneumonia, collapsed lungs and whatever cold or flu was passing through at the time. I spent much of my early life in hospitals and on many, many medications.

When my mother was prescribed medication for an infection, I refused breastfeeding (my tiny body *knew*!). I was subsequently given cow's milk and, as my mom puts it, "The cow's milk did not go well." Although cow's milk was later replaced by unpasteurized goat's milk from a nearby farm, I shudder to think of some of the other foods I was unwittingly fed throughout my childhood (slices of margarine, anyone?).

Back then, however, the effects of food on body systems weren't widely understood and my parents were actually told by one of my doctors that "food has nothing to do with her health issues." Fortunately, this made no sense to my mom, who'd watched me projectile vomit every dairy product I ingested and couldn't help but notice I wet the bed every time I ate kidney beans.

I'll probably never definitively trace my health issues back to any one food or medication. But we now know that cow's milk and gluten alone (not to mention the medications I was prescribed, including long-term corticosteroids and course after course of antibiotics) can damage gut linings and often negatively influence health in a number of significant ways.

Throughout my life, I experienced all kinds of food and environmental allergies. I dreaded each new set of scratch tests, which I endured on an annual basis for many years. I experienced a seemingly endless barrage of skin rashes, yeast infections, acne, never-ending mucous and, when I got older, periodic but severe lower back pain due to badly herniated discs. I went for weekly allergy shots, which I hated with a passion, and continued to get every cold or flu that came down the pike. In school, I was always the "sick kid." Later, as a commercial actor, I lived in near-constant, low-level anxiety about whether or not I'd be ill or have acne breakouts on my shoot dates. As a speech pathologist working in the public schools, I was exposed to a steady stream of students' coughs, sneezes and runny noses. My poor immune system was a mess, I was constantly on multiple medications, and I rarely experienced anything approaching actual good health.

Until my early thirties I dealt with my symptoms the Western medicine way: with medications. Even though these were never more than partially effective, in my family medicine and doctors were tantamount to God and were credited with the "miracle" that I had made it past infanthood alive. Of course I bought into all of this medicine-is-magic hook, line and sinker (*sometimes* it is) and just kept going with the pharmaceuticals. I knew nothing else.

Following many years of multiple asthma medications, my lung issues were finally under control with only occasional steroid use. Antibiotics continued to be prescribed to clear up recurrent respiratory infections—while at the same time allowing yeast infections to take over. After a failed course of Accutane (which resulted in temporary hair loss—yikes), my skin remained fairly clear of acne as long as I took three prescription medications and used several topical creams, which degraded the quality of my skin. To alleviate the agony of my lower back issues, my doctor prescribed stronger and stronger pain medications. Without birth control pills, my periods were irregular and I was a hormonal mess.

This regimen, as you can imagine, resulted in additional complications, side effects and long-term health risks. And it exhausted me.

At a certain point I recognized the futility of continuing down the path of lotions, potions and prescription medications. It became apparent that I'd come to the end of what my traditional doctors (as good and well-meaning as they were) could offer me.

Spurred on by pain and dissatisfaction with my health, I slowly shifted gears. I began to immerse myself in serious research and, more importantly, to apply what I learned to my life. I explored various therapies and made discoveries about the relationship between diet and health. I began to notice huge differences in the way I felt when I ate certain foods and eliminated others. I found, for example, that by decreasing processed sugars and eliminating dairy and grains (and subsequently gluten) from my diet, the stomach upsets, rashes and brain fog disappeared. Diet, I found, was indeed a critical key for me.

Those initial improvements fueled my desire to continue discovering which foods and food combinations supported thriving health. I amped up my research and experimentation while paying close attention to how my body responded to every intervention.

One thing became clear to me over the years: no one was going to do this for me but me, and no one *could*. I was the only one able to observe what felt right and what didn't.

Taking the Vegan Plunge

When I was about ten years old I sat at the dinner table, squinting at a chicken leg on my plate and noticing the bumps on its skin where the feathers had been removed. I glanced out our kitchen window to the chicken coop where my little flock of hens—my best friends—scratched and pecked their happy-chicken hearts out. "How can those birds outside be family," I wondered, "and this bird on my plate be food?" To eat them felt wrong to me, and I pushed away my plate in disgust.

Of course, I was only ten at the time, and despite this moment of clarity I soon went back to our typical family diet, meat and all.

When I began my nutritional research and experimentation phase in my thirties, I came across the vegan diet. My son had recently become a vegan, and the more I learned, the more I loved the idea. I had never lost my feeling of kinship with non-human animals, though it certainly did get pushed to the side when it came to my dietary choices, as it does for many of us. I gradually began decreasing the presence of meat in my diet and focused instead on seafood and "disguised" meats, such as shredded pork in enchiladas.

Then I enrolled in a degree program in environmental studies. As soon as I became aware of the lurid details of factory farming, all bets were off. I stopped eating all animals and animal products except fish, until one fateful night in my Resources Management class when I sat in the back and bawled through a film about the horrors of commercial fishing practices. No more fish for me!

For a while, anyway.

Some of my research had led me to the misguided belief that I needed fish to stay healthy, so I continued to consume fish here and there for some time before realizing there are whole communities of people who *never* have access to fish and do just fine without it. Ultimately I gave up fish and went completely vegan.

With the exception of my son, who shared with me his own wisdom, research and support, my family and friends thought I'd finally gone off the deep end. I wasn't swayed. Why not? Because soon after starting to eat completely animal-free foods, not only did I notice significant improvements in my physical health, I also felt something else click into place: *the sensation of my actions aligning with my heart.*

Integrity.

Authenticity.

Connection.

Aha! What a fantastic feeling!

My Intro to Raw Vegan

I felt wonderful on so many levels after transitioning to a vegan diet. However, due to a few remaining, nagging health issues I continued to keep an ear cocked for any additional helpful diet tweaks.

Enter *raw* vegan foods.

We'll explore the raw food diet in great depth in this book, but essentially going "raw vegan" means eating mainly unprocessed and uncooked foods, and no meat or animal-derived products, such as eggs or dairy. When I first heard about the raw foods diet during a period of recovery from serious back issues, the concept seemed ridiculous and over the top—a bridge too far. How could I give up the delicious vegan scones I'd finally mastered? And seriously, I'd already made so many changes in my diet that another big one seemed like overkill.

But everywhere I looked, there it was: the raw food diet.

You know when you get a new car and suddenly start to notice the same make and model everywhere you go? That's what happened to me with raw food. It just wouldn't leave me alone!

Back then, due to herniated discs and excruciating back pain, I spent a lot of time at my chiropractor's office, and his waiting room was well-stocked with books on health. It was there I discovered and devoured *The Coconut Oil Miracle*[1] and *Green for Life.*[2] I subsequently added coconut oil and green smoothies to my diet and began to look and feel better than ever. Fairly quickly I noticed I needed to use my asthma medications less frequently as well.

One day I noticed a flier advertising a talk by raw food "guru"

Tonya Zavasta. I'd never heard of her, but I felt drawn to this presentation and signed up, dragging my son along with me.

We sat through her presentation in awed silence. At the end of the talk, I turned to my son and whispered, "I'm doing this."

Tonya was in her fifties but didn't look a day over thirty-five. I'm not gonna lie—that's what tipped the scales for me at first. Not the pain relief or the phenomenal health benefits, but the vanity.

I bought Tonya's books, followed her plan for transitioning to raw foods—and never looked back.

Transitioning to a Raw Vegan Diet

Right off the bat I came face to face with an all-too-familiar problem: many people thought I was even *more* insane than when I'd gone vegan!

The general message I got from the peanut gallery was that my health would deteriorate. I heard everything from "You'll lose your hair!" (which *really* freaked me out) to warnings about my skin conditions worsening and assurances that I'd become emaciated and suffer from untold nutritional deficiencies and their resulting disorders. (I might add that in retrospect I realize none of these naysayers had ever actually tried the raw vegan lifestyle.)

Now, from the vantage point of someone who's done the research and lived the raw vegan lifestyle for many years, it's clear that these dire predictions didn't have any solid rationale behind them. But at the time, I shared some of these concerns.

This lifestyle was completely new to me, and there wasn't much hard and fast research out there about eating exclusively raw vegan. But there *was* an increasing body of scientific evidence supporting the benefits of a plant-based diet, as well as information that laid bare the negative health and environmental effects of the Standard American Diet (see Chapter Three: What We Won't Be Eating). I decided this was enough for me to go on, and I dove in, fear and all.

The first few months on raw food I counted calories, studied nutrients and *stressed out.* I met with my doctor for baseline lab tests and continued to have them rechecked along the way.

Despite these safety measures, I still felt alone and a little afraid. The nagging fear persisted: could I eat enough calories and get enough nutrients, long-term, to sustain my health? I remember occasionally waking up in the middle of the night in an honest-to-goodness panic, thinking that maybe everyone else was right and I really was doing something crazy. I often felt I was charting my own path through the jungle.

Along the way, though, I found signposts and maps. In addition to Tonya Zavasta, these included the work of people like Philip McCluskey, David Wolfe, Markus Rothkranz, Alyssa Cohen, Raw Matt, Storm Talifaro, Natasha St. Michael and Juliano Brotman. I absorbed oodles of blogs, videos, the occasional coaching session and a gaggle of raw food "un-cook" books. After attending her classes at local food co-ops, I also became friends with Brooke Preston, a supportive and inspirational raw food chef in my home town. I'm forever grateful to all of these folks whose experience and willingness to share themselves and their wisdom illuminated the path before me.

These invaluable resources helped me further educate myself. They also served as much-needed emotional support along the way and offered advice and practical tips regarding equipment, supplies and recipes. With the help of my "virtual team" I began to get the hang of it.

Learning to Thrive

Almost immediately I noticed an increase in energy, sounder sleep, and a clearer mental state. My back pain diminished and then disappeared. I began to experience what the word "thriving" truly means. I was looking and feeling better and better—and I was happy. This lifestyle felt *right* to me.

My lab tests continued to come back with increasingly positive results. My doctor, initially reluctant to support this new lifestyle, finally shook her head and admitted, "Whatever you're doing, keep doing it. You're healthier than anyone else I see." Eventually, she began refusing to perform the routine blood tests as frequently as I'd been requesting them, noting that unless I changed my diet, there was no reason to keep checking: I was officially incredibly healthy.

When your Western medical doctor tells you *that,* you know you're really onto something.

I was ecstatic. None of my earlier fears had come true. Rather than deteriorating, my health—and my life—continued to improve day by day.

Although I already knew even without the lab tests that my body was happy, those early results were a great confirmation for me—and for my family and friends, who respected this scientific stamp of approval. The lab results helped quell our fears and encouraged me to keep trucking along, trying this, testing that, listening to my body, and reading and researching my new path to health.

What I eventually discovered was that after a period of detoxification, my body knew what to eat all on its own. I stopped counting calories and stressing out. I had returned to the inherent wisdom of my true self. It had been inside me all along.

Just as yours is within you.

A friend once remarked to me after a healthy lunch, "You have a very lucky body. Not many people listen to and take care of themselves like you do."

The truth is, I'm thankful and honored to be aware enough and able to do so now. This wasn't always the case. That baby, whose body knew to get rid of the dairy products, had become a woman who'd gone numb and forgotten how to listen to her body's signals.

I know better now. I listen, and my body rewards me with excellent health, quick healing when I do get sick, clarity, and the energy of a twelve year old.

Our bodies are incredible, unbelievable, fantastic gifts. To live in gratitude and care for them to the best of our abilities (and to fully and authentically LIVE our lives) is for me the only proper response to such a gift. Raw food has been an absolute boon for my health, and has allowed my body to resume the work it does so well: balancing and healing itself, and allowing me to live the truth of who I am, largely unencumbered by discomfort, lethargy and disease.

Having lived as a raw vegan for over a decade now, no one who knows me argues against my diet or lifestyle anymore. It's clearly working for me. It's hard to argue with someone who's glowing, happy, energetic and free of her once-chronic health conditions.

In short, the proof is in the raw vegan chia pudding!

Part I

Why Go Raw?

Chapter One

The Raw Food Manifesto

R aw food is now effortlessly integrated into my daily life. But as I've described, it wasn't always this way.

My aim in this book is to save you more time than you can imagine by sparing you much of the uncertainty, frustration, fear, and trial and error I went through. I want to get you straight to the good stuff: a simple, healthy, self-connected, raw way of life. Pura vida! Within these pages I provide all the information you need to get started, including simple meal structures you can use as-is or get creative with. I'll show you how to create nutritious and tasty green smoothies and all of my raw menu basics. And although this isn't a cookbook per se (there are plenty of great ones out there), I also share several easy, fantastic recipes from a friend: world-renowned raw vegan chef Ronald Russell of the award-winning SunCafe Organic in Los Angeles.

In the Preface I shared with you what raw vegan food did for me. In this next section we're going to look at what it can do for you—and the planet. Our dietary choices, especially when considered en masse, impact Mother Earth in a multitude of ways. On an individual level, eating a raw vegan diet can activate an empowering force within you that supports optimal health, including (but not limited to!) assisting in maintaining a healthy weight, reducing inflammation, improving energy levels and immunity, lowering blood pressure, increasing heart health and improving digestion. These changes reduce susceptibility to a wide range of related issues as well, such as obesity, diabetes, stroke, heart disease, asthma, allergies, hormonal imbalances, fibromyalgia, accelerated aging and more. The list goes on and on.

As mentioned however, this book is about much more than just physical health and how to create tasty and nutritious raw meals. My intention is to share that important information and instruction within the broader context of something even more critical: reconnection with our community and our world at large through reconnection with *ourselves*.

The Problem: Disconnection

As a species, we've lost our way on many fronts. We have been misdirected, distracted and overstimulated. We've forgotten how we fit into the web of life. Most of us no longer understand ourselves as part of nature. In many ways we perceive ourselves as separate from the natural environment.

It certainly doesn't help that over the past hundred years or so we've become almost completely disconnected from the sources of our food. In fact, we've altered what we consider food to be. We've moved away from whole, natural ingredients and become used to eating refined and processed food-like "products." Our physical systems often no longer recognize what we're eating.

One consequence is that we have become disconnected from *ourselves*. We have lost contact with the intuitive wisdom of our bodies and forgotten who we truly are. We're told we need to go outside ourselves to find out what we should be eating. We consult so-called "experts" via celebrities, advertising, books, articles and television shows rather than look to the *real* experts on our bodies: our bodies themselves!

Ask yourself: does a deer need to be told what to eat, or even have to think about it? Or a platypus, or a squirrel? No.

And neither do we.

Our bodies already possess an intuitive "knowing" regarding which foods to choose to support optimal health and well-being. The problem is that in our modern world we allow overthinking and marketing to override this inherent wisdom. We wait for "scientific proof" that eating berries is healthy for us before we're willing to try them. We ignore whatever proof our bodies—if we would only *listen* to them—offer us on a moment-by-moment basis.

The quality of the food we eat compounds the confusion: any signals our inner voice sends us must make their way through the interference of brain fog, chemical addictions, low energy and often poor health resulting from our diets. We're frequently stressed-out, overworked and used to making food choices based on convenience rather than what our bodies need. We've disconnected and lost touch.

Reconnection — and Revolution

I ♥ Raw explores how this disconnection occurs, but more importantly it shows how we may be inspired, through the delicious path of nutrition, to *re*connect with ourselves and the world around us. By reconnecting to ourselves, we can regain access to our intuition and to the freedom of simply *knowing* what to eat.

Steve Gagné observes that, "the food folklore of our 'unscientific' past finally is reemerging as the foundation of healing, and what was condemned yesterday as blind superstition is reappearing as today's validated scientific fact."[3]

Imagine everything you eat being seamlessly in sync with the rhythm of your existence, so much so that choosing and preparing foods requires little effort. Next imagine that eating this way supports the health and well-being of the planet as well. Finally, imagine knowing and feeling that your food choices are so absolutely *right* that cravings and old habits no longer exert any power over you.

So yes, *I ♥ Raw* is about raw food, but it's also about empowerment, authenticity, reconnection, transformation and love. It's about realizing the freedom you already possess. And, in a very real way, it's about revolution.

The kind of revolution that emancipates us from:

- The manipulative tentacles of marketing

- The lack of power we feel over our health and food choices

- The oppression of social convention

- The chains of physical aches, pains and dis-ease that most of us accept as part of daily life and aging

This is the kind of revolution that supports reconnection with:

- Clarity

- Optimal conditions for health and healing

- Trust in our own bodies

- The freedom to choose food based on what our bodies want and need rather than what we're told we should eat

- The power to vote with our feet—and our dollars—for a world where we care for and support each other and treat ourselves, the environment and all life with respect and compassion.

When we reconnect to and align our actions with our intuitive wisdom, we inspire others to do the same—creating an exponential expansion toward wholeness. This impulse toward healing on a large scale must be a grassroots effort; we can no longer wait for others to do it for us. WE are the leaders of this revolution, and we have never been in greater need of it than we are right now.

It's Now or Never

Reconnection is not a luxury. It's literally a matter of life or death for ourselves, our fellow creatures and our environment. The survival of our species and other life forms depends upon our reconnection with our bodies and our hearts. Compassionate action is required to reverse the damage we've wrought and to create sustainable, life-centric ways of being in the world. We are at a critical tipping point. On the one hand we have health and hope. On the other we have destruction, degeneration and despair. The outside world (our home) mirrors our collective inner state, and neither is in great shape at the moment.

The barrage of pollution we're faced with has been implicated in everything from plummeting fertility rates and rising disease incidence to climate change and autism rates. Processed foods, the lifestyle degradation we experience daily (stress, inattention, etc.), the harmful chemicals in our food and environment, and exposure to electromagnetic fields and radiation are just a few of the culprits, along with many other aspects of the standard American lifestyle. As MIT researcher Stefanie Seneff, Ph.D., points out, if we wait for our government to make the necessary changes for us, there is little hope.[4]

Change must come from individuals making different choices—choices that come from the heart, and not just from the pocketbook. What will be our bottom line? Money or life?

To make true and informed choices, we need to reconnect with our *own* hearts.

So let's get real and *raw.*

Getting Back to Raw

The word "raw" in the phrase "raw food lifestyle" means much more to me than just "uncooked." For me, "raw" connotes authenticity on every level: in relationships, career, spirituality, physicality and every other aspect of existence. Living a raw lifestyle means being honest, genuine and connected with who we truly are.

The healing journey back to intuition and wholeness is, in a sense, the journey many of us make over the course of our lives. If we are on a path of awakening, we unlearn our programming bit by bit and become more of who we truly are in every moment. Each individual's authentic reconnection inspires more connections, and before you know it, we're all healing. Healthy habits are just as contagious as unhealthy ones. Yet we are each responsible for our own reconnection. No one else can do it for us.

In my first book, *Guided by Your Own Stars,* I offered fundamental how-to's on the basics of reconnecting with the true self, dissolving self-imposed limitations and realizing personal freedom. In *I ♥ Raw* we'll do something similar, only this time in the context of our current food culture.

Why do we make the choices we do when it comes to food, and how do they impact us and the planet? How do outside influences like advertising and scientific studies play a role in defining our diets? And if we're unhappy, or at least confused about where we find ourselves in relation to diet, how can we free ourselves from the perceived tyranny of food to make lasting, healthy changes?

In *I ♥ Raw* I propose that the path to true health gets us back in touch with our body's own internal GPS (our intuitive wisdom), allowing it to guide us to food choices that nurture spirit, body, community, natural ecosystems and the planet.

The Power of Raw Food

The cleanliness, simplicity and pure energy of raw vegan food can be a powerful ally in our return to wholeness.

Never underestimate the power of food. The condition of our bodies and minds has everything to do with how we experience our lives. What we eat profoundly affects our state of consciousness. Thanks in part to poor food choices, most people are so used to a degraded quality of experience that they assume it's just how things have to be.

In his inspired book, *Food Energetics,* Steve Gagné notes, "Dining at nature's table as directly as possible—without agribiz and high-tech, genetically altering intermediaries—is a sensible way of reconnecting yourself with the earth."[5] We all have the power to do this, to reconnect with our wise, authentic selves and return to optimal conditions for health and healing. By applying common sense and reconnecting with our inherent wisdom, we create a space for our bodies to communicate to us what they need—and then we simply respond to this knowing.

As in all arenas of life, when the mind becomes a faithful servant of the knowing of the body and the life force, health and clarity return. Released from food confusion and angst, we are free to make the right choices for ourselves in the moment.

Raw food, whether used as a short-term cleanse, a month-long reset or a long-term lifestyle, is an amazing way to realign with nature, inner self, true health—and life itself.

What Will I Eat?

For those new to raw foods, the term "raw vegan" simply means consuming primarily whole, real and unprocessed/minimally processed foods free of animal flesh and animal products, with nothing heated over 118 degrees Fahrenheit. Although raw vegan options include uncooked fruits, vegetables, nuts and seeds, this does NOT mean you'll just be eating salads every day! Believe it or not, within these simple categories you'll find potentially infinite variety.

The flip side of *What will I eat?* is equally relevant: *What* won't *I eat?* The world of raw vegan food is a world away from the Standard American Diet and even from what many health conscious folks are familiar with.

We'll look at this question in depth in Chapter Two. For now, I'll just reiterate that as a society we've largely forgotten what real food is. We often rely on premade dishes in which any remaining original, whole ingredients are irradiated, pasteurized, bleached, fortified and otherwise processed beyond recognition into what manufacturers call "food products."

In a word (and often in the scientific sense of the word), important, naturally-occurring elements in the foods we consume are *denatured*. With raw foods, we're re-naturing; we're returning to nature, and in the process returning to our own true natures.

Won't It Be Overwhelming?

The process of making changes in our lives tends to bring us face to face with ourselves. Going raw vegan is likely to introduce us to a host of our own untested beliefs, such as:

- It's too expensive to eat right!

- I don't have the time to make healthy meals!

- I can't give up cheese and bread.

- There's so much confusing information out there; I'm giving up and eating whatever I feel like!

- I'm going to die anyway! What's the use of changing anything?

- I NEED (x, y, or z food) to survive.

We'll examine these issues in more detail in the next chapter, but suffice it to say that it's not your fault if past efforts to eat healthy felt like navigating an obstacle course. Scaling the walls of scientific studies, wading through advertising campaigns, decoding chemical names and food labels, wrestling with side effects and fighting through a never-ending deluge of diet books—all that would make anyone feel crazy, confused and ready to give up!

When we begin making different food choices, we often feel bereft of our go-to comfort foods, or even of staple food items we've come to rely on daily, such as eggs or milk.

The process of rediscovering vibrant health for yourself can involve a bit of a learning curve—or more accurately, an *un*learning curve. Even so, you might be surprised at how simple it can be. I promise, after you get the hang of it you'll wonder why eating this way ever seemed like such a big deal.

How "Easy" *Is* It?

Once upon a time I purchased an "easy" twenty-one-day raw food cleanse for a friend, sight unseen. Any "easy" raw cleanse would do, right? How could you mess *that* up?

I was about to find out. He called me soon after it arrived.

"Christy, um, it looks a little . . . overwhelming."

I could hear the hesitation in his voice and assured him, "It *said* 'easy'!"

Then I took a look at it, and . . . yikes!

I'd been eating raw vegan for years, and it was overwhelming to *me*. Any plan, cleanse or diet that requires the eater to wrangle with a shopping list longer than their couch and twice as expensive is not, by my definition, "easy." As far as I'm concerned, if everyday recipes include more than a few readily available ingredients, take more than a few minutes to prepare, require über-expensive specialty ingredients, necessitate creating several different dishes each day or consist only of salads—they're fails!

I advised my friend to ditch that "easy" cleanse program. If I had been a newbie raw foodie myself I probably would have thrown it out the window and ordered a pizza!

Why This Book Is Different

Just like that cleanse, many raw food how-to books claim to be easy guides to the raw food lifestyle but in reality are complicated and overwhelming. Worse, they can actually discourage well-intentioned folks from healthy eating in general.

I'm not suggesting that fully transitioning from the Standard

American Diet to a raw food diet (if that's your intention) is effortless. But it *is* extremely doable. And if you're looking for a truly honest take on the raw food lifestyle from someone who's walking the talk, you're in the right place. I can show you how to make eating raw *truly* easy.

There are some specific issues we tend to run into when transitioning to a raw vegan diet. When I first started out, I stumbled into quite a few of these potholes. One of the reasons I wrote this book was to help you avoid those same potholes, and maybe a few others as well. The less reinventing of the wheel we need to do, the better.

At the same time, I promise not to pull any punches. Eating raw is simple for me *now*, but it wasn't always. If you're like most folks making any major shift, you'll find change is often exciting, sometimes daunting, periodically confusing and possibly exhausting. I'm here to hold your hand through all this: you can do it!

Your transition to a raw food lifestyle will take some patience, time, and perhaps even a little money if you invest in equipment. I'll show you how to do it all with minimal difficulty and expense. Once you're set up you'll be able to glide on your own, with no more effort (and perhaps even less) than it takes to prepare and cook food the way you're probably used to doing now.

Everything here really *is* easy. Ingredients, recipes and food prep aside, at its core, this book is about remembering that *your body already knows what to eat.* We just have to remember how to become aware of its wisdom, and listen to it.

How I Define "Easy"

I love good food. I want simple, healthy and *tasty* food that's quick to shop for and prepare. I need a basic overall structure to my eating plan, one that takes very little thought, time or effort. If it's not easy, I won't do it. Period. It has to work for me and my complex life, or it's out.

With my raw food lifestyle, I have all that and more, and I'm so excited to share it with you!

You can go all-out-gourmet with raw foods, just as with any other type of cuisine, and that's where many raw chefs shine. I'm not a chef, and I rarely get fancy with my food, but if you're looking to give raw foods a try in a way that's doable for the average person and sustainable for the long haul, I'm your girl.

Prepare yourself to engage in a new kind of food experience, one that will free up energy and serve as a catalyst for healthy transformation in every area of your life.

The How and the Why

If you'd like to get straight into the "how-to" portion of the book and come back to read about the "why" later, be my guest. Feel free to read the chapters in any order you like. To skip to the how-to section, jump to Section II: The Nuts and Bolts.

However, if you're interested in soaking up some of the behind-the-scenes info before you dive in—and possibly discovering some additional motivation for your journey—please enjoy the following sections. They explore my philosophy of the raw food lifestyle, the psychology of food choices and some of the many benefits of a raw vegan diet.

Chapter Two

A Deeper Look into Food Decisions: The New "Normal"

What's become normal food for us as a culture is anything but natural.

The term "normal" indicates that something's been culturally agreed upon. It tells us that's how things are "supposed to be," or at least how most people do or see things. While "normal" often implies "acceptable," we've arrived at a tipping point where it's becoming harder and harder to ignore the fact that the Standard American Diet, though widely accepted as normal, is quite literally killing us.

Poor diet is a major contributor to chronic disease and death in the United States, including coronary heart disease, diabetes, hyperlipidemia, and stroke.[6] The Centers for Disease Control (CDC) statistics from 2018 reported that roughly 42 percent of Americans are obese.[7] Obesity alone increases the risk of multiple health conditions, including:

- Coronary heart disease, stroke, and high blood pressure
- Type 2 diabetes

- Certain types of cancer, such as endometrial, breast and colon cancer
- High total cholesterol/triglycerides
- Liver and gallbladder disease
- Sleep apnea and respiratory problems
- Degeneration of cartilage and osteoarthritis
- Reproductive health complications, such as erectile dysfunction and infertility
- Mental health conditions

The over-processed, over-chemicalized, over-salted, over-sweetened foods we're marketed take years off of our lives and undermine our quality of life as well. This is an important consideration. Even if we don't extend the *number* of years we live, there is an immense difference between living a full eighty years in excellent health versus spending the last twenty of those in a medicated haze and downward spiral of discomfort, pain and disease.

For many people today, this slow decline has become the new normal. How can we be effective powerhouses of passion, doing wonderful work in the world, if our attention is consumed by "normal" aches and pains, let alone chronic disease?

Please note that while in this section I share my own research and personal observations with you and hope that much of what I've included here will resonate with you, I also want to remind you that I am not trained in food psychology. If you're struggling with eating disorders or other mental health issues, I encourage you to include the support of trained professionals to help guide you on your journey to wellness.

So with that said, let's dig a little deeper into the forces that influence our dietary choices.

Food and Power

Can food have any power over you?

Yes and no.

Try this little thought experiment. Imagine setting a bunch of grapes and a bag of chips on your countertop. Stare intently at both.

How likely is it that either item jumps into your mouth on its own? Or compels you to reach out and force feed it to yourself?

I'm pretty sure what you'll find is that they just sit there, side by side, being grapes and chips; they don't wield any inherent psychic power to compel you to devour them. In fact, if we go a little deeper, drop their labels and look at them with complete clarity, we can see that they're just objects sitting on the countertop, no different from your cell phone or a magazine. Still . . .

We typically *do* find ourselves compelled to eat one over the other (usually the chips) and often feel that we have frustratingly little control over these choices. Why is that? Why do so many of us make choices that can contribute to our being overweight, sick, tired and depressed—even when we try not to?

Most of us are generally aware of which foods are healthy and which are not. Despite many forces attempting to sell us junk food, we all know that eating an apple is far healthier than eating a donut. And yet we continue to consume unhealthy foods in the face of all the health complications listed above.

Clearly, this is one of those "simple but not easy" issues.

Unless we address some of the underlying reasons we bypass healthy food for junk, we'll stumble before we get out of the gate. Bringing the motivations for unhealthy choices to light creates a scenario in which we can no longer make those choices without awareness.

This is important: without awareness there is no choice. In the light of awareness, we are often empowered to make different choices.

These new choices may feel uncomfortable at first. But as we become aware of our misperceptions and reconnect with our own intuitive knowing, our choices align with our body's wisdom. We create new habits.

We typically gravitate toward what we're used to, and it's time to get used to food choices that create vibrant health rather than disconnection, pain and disease.

This is where our power lies: not in food or willpower, but in our ability to connect with and act from what our bodies already know.

Why We Eat What We Eat — and How to Start Changing It

Let's discuss some common motivators behind our food choices and consider how to upgrade those choices.

Confusion/Information Overload

With all of the studies and books and gurus (not to mention social media, our family and friends) out there dispensing conflicting information about what we should and shouldn't eat, it's no wonder we often become overwhelmed and even despondent about making healthy food choices. There are legitimate questions to ask about this data stream. Was a study funded by a corporate food giant or other invested party? How do we even find that out? Why is coffee good for you one day and bad the next? How much broccoli is too much? Is that food "expert" concerned more about your health or making a buck? In short: what's really reliable?

I'm not advocating burying our heads in the sand and pooh-poohing books, articles, others' experiences or scientific data—far from it. But I'd like to reiterate that whatever sources of information we consider, *the most reliable health expert will be our own bodies.*

So how *do* we make sense of all the information out there? Here are a few points to consider:

- Dr. Howard Jacobson, co-author of *Whole: Rethinking the Science of Nutrition,*[8] points out that science tends to take the tiniest slice of reality and dive deeply into it. Due to this "trees for the forest" approach, in addition to the inability to test for the millions of synergistic effects that occur when we ingest a single bite of food, we can't often get a holistic understanding from this reductionist viewpoint. On top of that, we are only privy to studies that get funding, and where that funding comes from is an important factor in analyzing the data.

- When an author writes a diet book, it often promotes a specific plan or set of products that may be great for some but not for others. It might not even be great for *anyone*!

- Food blogs and articles are often created with a specific agenda in mind, or written by people with little to no actual nutritional knowledge or education.

It's clear that we need a big-picture, commonsense approach to deciding how to eat, rather than an unending and hopeless effort to define the perfect diet in terms of this or that minute aspect or detail, such as individual nutrients, calorie count or glycemic index.

So what IS the big picture?

The answer is much simpler than you may think. The 2015–2020 Dietary Guidelines for Americans, informed by a group of the nation's top health experts who spent two years analyzing nutritional data, recommend eating more plants and less meat.[9] Even though there are troubling issues in terms of corporate interest influence on the Food and Drug Administration's (FDA) final diet recommendations, one thing that is agreed upon in most current food science research is that optimal health involves a varied, plant-based diet, which can drastically reduce and even reverse many health problems.[10]

Convenience/Availability

Another significant factor in food choice is how easily we can acquire, prepare and consume our food. This is often one of the simpler motivations to address, though it will fluctuate depending on where you live. Isn't it crazy that in some places it might be easier to find a processed snack cake than a simple salad?

Fortunately, healthy, organic, whole foods are becoming more and more available in the United States and abroad. Several online grocery stores in the U.S. offer organic produce and other items at reduced rates, making access to these items simple no matter where one is located. Throughout this book, I'll delve more deeply into methods for locating fresh, healthy foods, but what I'd like to discuss in this section is *effort*.

If you've patronized the same grocery stores or fast food joints for years, it can be a little daunting to think about trying something new. But "new" may be just what eating healthy requires. It may be easier and more convenient to go through a fast food drive-thru than locate a new grocery store, find a parking spot, get out of your car and navigate unfamiliar aisles. I get it; I used to frequent a few fast food places myself for just this reason. So here's where the effort comes in.

If your normal daily routines consistently result in unhealthy food choices, maybe it's time to switch it up. For one thing, if you're really serious about getting healthy, simply cross fast food off your list of viable options. Sure, some offer salads or sliced fruit, but consider:

You're paying good money for run-of-the-mill choices.

Dressings and dipping sauces can double or triple the calorie count of your "healthy" option, while adding sugar and salt.

Ingredients tend to be low quality, cheap and nutrient-light.

Unless it's organic, you're also most likely ingesting pesticides, preservatives and other chemicals as a side dish. Blech.

In short, save "healthy" fast-food salads and other menu options for travel or for when you're desperate and truly don't have time to pop into a grocery store. Packing a bag of nuts or seeds in your purse, briefcase or car will help avoid the "desperately hungry" scenario.

So, to create new habits, here's how to start.

First, find a grocery store that's fairly close to you.

Next, locate its organic produce and nuts and seeds (often found in bulk) sections.

Finally, buy anything you want to from these sections.

Period.

You've just considerably upgraded the quality of your nutritional intake over that of the average American.

Later in the book we'll be talking more about what to do with those foods. For now, just start redefining what "convenient" means for you, and begin creating new food-finding habits. Because you know what's *really* inconvenient? Obesity, cancer and heart disease.

Habit/Tradition

Most of what we eat has everything to do with what we're used to. As the saying goes, we are creatures of habit.

The most familiar choices also tend to be the most comfortable, so that's right where we go, wearing deeper and deeper grooves into our old food habits. Whether it's picking up items at the grocery store on auto-pilot, ordering take-out from a favorite pizza place or repeatedly booking reservations at the same old restaurant, food habits can begin to feel like old friends—but many times they're not.

Examining our food habits can be extremely enlightening. Take a few moments now and think about your food go-to's. Where do you go to get food on a daily basis, whether at home, at work, on a date or social outing, or when traveling?

Now take a long look at these habits through the eyes of "happy" versus "unhappy" body choices. From this fresh perspective, which items or places can you simply cross off your mental go-to list?

If you find some favorite hangouts on the list that you just don't want to give up, could you at least switch to healthier choices on their menus? Could you ask the chef to prepare something sans this or that, or with added veggies? What options exist to up the nutrient value and decrease the junk factor?

Start exploring healthier options to replace the old, unhealthy ones. Maybe make it an adventure to try a new restaurant, store or snack food once a week. Begin to examine and adjust unhealthy habits one by one. As we move along with the book, I'll suggest lots of ideas for how to create healthy food options on your own and crowd out those old, unhealthy ones.

You may also notice more deeply ingrained habits on your list, perhaps tied to specific cultural, religious or familial customs. We often call these traditions. While some folks don't identify with any actual traditional foods of this nature, many unhealthy American foods have become *de facto* "traditional" fare. Think about pizza, hamburgers and fried chicken. Or a hot dog and a beer at a sporting event. And can you get through movie night without popcorn, soda or ice cream?

Just because a food seems normal or is widely available does not mean it's healthy. Recognizing this can go a long way towards helping you make better choices.

Granted, if your family prepares traditional foods at holidays, this can be tough. But it doesn't have to be a big deal either. Something eaten once a year is not likely to be a problem. It's our overall *habits,* the foods we eat on a daily basis, that create our state of overall health.

Take a look at what you're eating and why. Are there staple items your mother or grandmother used to make? Many traditional foods were originally prepared using healthy, whole-food ingredients that have slowly been switched out for processed, cheap replacements. Processed foods have only been around a little over a hundred years and those whole, healthy foods are just waiting for you to rediscover them again.

It's important to note here that creating new habits is a very powerful way to reprogram subconscious "recordings". No matter what your underlying reason is for continuing to choose unhealthy food when your intention is otherwise, employing the tool of habit creation can break the chains of these old subconscious motivations.[11]

Seasonal Pull

We tend to desire heavier, warmer foods in autumn and winter, and lighter, cooler foods in the spring and summer. Purchasing ingredients from a farmers' market or ordering from a local farm will ensure you're getting some of the seasonal fare your body is craving without falling into the pit of often over-sweetened, salted and processed go-to's. Creating healthy soups or warm drinks can easily fit the bill when the weather's chilly, just as selecting fresh, juicy fruits like watermelon in the summer can satisfy the need for cool, refreshing foods.

Thirst

This one's really simple. Oftentimes we mistake thirst for hunger. If you find yourself feeling hungry at odd times, try downing a big glass of water before eating or snacking. This is an easy experiment you can use to check in with your body. Just drink first and then see how you feel. Even if you discover that you really are hungry after your glass of water, this one simple step can create a mental pause and allow you to consciously choose a healthier snack or meal rather than automatically reaching for a familiar, less healthy go-to standby.

Advertising/Association

We've been sold a lot of "goods" (now *there's* a clever marketing term if I ever heard one) since the advent of advertising, and a fantasy version of health is one of them. I'm talking about the seemingly healthy people we see in media campaigns of all kinds, trumpeting the benefits of everything from the latest miracle food, personal product or pharmaceutical drug to cars, home security systems and retirement accounts. Everyone's noticed, but maybe some have never really pondered the fact that almost everyone in advertisements appears happy and healthy.

I've worked as a commercial actor for over a decade, and I'll tell you a little secret that everyone already knows: the vast majority of marketing is fake!

You may ask, "Why does advertising exist if everyone knows it's fake?" Answer: Because it still works! On some level, we still believe the images that enter our field of vision at the rate of up to 5,000 ads per day.[12]

Images that pair the appearance of "health" with a product are often enticing to us, if only on a subconscious level. But the truth is, that newly arthritis-free gardening granny pretending to swallow that nifty new drug is probably forty-five years old and doesn't have arthritis.

Likewise, the sassy mom serving colorfully-packaged, sugary fruit drinks to her happy and healthy family is really just an actress who may never have seen the product until the day of the shoot (I've been that T.V. mom dozens of times). Her peppy appearance is the result of youth and hours of professional hair, makeup, wardrobe and editing work. Keeping themselves looking good for the camera is often a big part of what commercial actors get paid for.

Put simply, the keys to marketing are aspirational characters and situations. Advertisers want viewers to *want* to be like the characters they've fabricated: happy, healthy and attractive. How do you accomplish that? By purchasing their product, of course!

Nothing about most advertising is real; it's all lighting, makeup, packaging and a well-thought-out, legally-proofed script. Don't buy into it. When ads come on, look away. Floss your teeth, take your dishes to the kitchen, play with your dog, write a gratitude list—do anything but stay glued to commercials.

We want to begin reducing the effects of outside influences on our choices and start listening to our own bodies. With very few exceptions, advertisers don't care about us or our health. Advertising on television, billboards and the Internet is there to make a buck—your health be damned. The less marketing you expose yourself to, the better.

On the flip side, you'd have to live in a cave to get away from it all; advertising is ubiquitous, insidious and often nearly invisible. Perhaps the best approach is simply to become aware of how it has infiltrated our lives and remember its purpose: making money by manipulating the consumer into thinking they need product x, y or z to be healthy. Take back your power from these companies by tuning into your body and finding what you *really* need.

Food as Substitution[13]

Food often feels easier to control than what's going on in our relationships, careers or emotional lives. Life can feel overwhelming, scary and out of control, so we sometimes look to control what we feel we *do* have some say over, such as our food choices. This can lead to substituting *food* satiety (feeling satisfied or comfortably full) for satiety in other areas of our lives.

It's an odd trick of transference between emotional and physical needs, but sometimes eating a donut can temporarily fill an emotional void. Food can act as a calming agent, incite a feeling of anxiety, make us sleepy or energize us. It can also serve to provide us with a sense of connection to others, if food (or a specific food or food group) was used in this way in our families. Though not widely recognized, food is one way we self-medicate and regulate our internal state.

Feeling anxious or out of control can lead to using food to suppress emotions rather than address difficult issues head-on. After all, addressing emotional issues and other challenges requires an awareness of what we're avoiding in the first place. It might be more appealing at first to get the immediate satisfaction of a rich meal or other substitute.

In a non-food example from my own experience, for years I moved from house to house on an annual basis. Instead of addressing what I really wanted to change (my job) I altered my living environment. It took me years to realize I was substituting moving for doing the scary, hard work of creating a satisfying work life. But after finally making changes in the areas I needed to address, I lost the overwhelming desire to move as frequently.

This kind of behavior doesn't mean we're lazy, dumb or unmotivated, so don't use it as an excuse to beat yourself up. It's actually an ingenious coping mechanism! But ultimately these substitutions don't lead us toward what we really want in our lives, including connection, health and alignment.

Taking an honest look at what's missing from the life experience you desire can be a powerful tool in remedying the situation. It can lead to actually making the desired changes instead of suppressing desires with food. The help of a life/health coach or other professional may be invaluable here, but to get started right away, try a simple exercise.

If you find you're clinging to a particular food, finish this sentence and see if anything helpful comes up for you: "I'm not ready to let go of this food [or eating habit] because it makes me feel _____."

What comes up for you? Do you "need" that slice of cake after a stressful day at work? Is a frothy, sugary coffee drink really the only way you can wake up in the morning? Or do even deeper reasons rise up from your subconscious?

Getting to the root of what you may be replacing or avoiding with food is probably the most important factor in dealing with food substitutions. But even before you do that, here are some practical ideas for replacing or interrupting emotional eating patterns with healthy choices:

- Crowd out: This simply means adding an abundance of healthy foods to your diet so that you fill up on these and don't have room for unhealthy choices. Literally crowding out unhealthy snacks with healthy ones in your cupboards and fridge can be a supportive strategy as well.

- Slow down: With most of us tending to multitask while we eat (myself included!), slowing down and becoming present to our food can be a game-changer. The idea is to "re-throne" food and the process of eating to its rightful status of a sacred practice, and thus to reinstate a positive relationship with eating. At the very least, taking a little more time to enjoy your meals will go a long way toward mindful consumption.

- Limit your consumption of unhealthy foods. Enjoying one cookie is a world away from eating the whole bag.

- Choose more high-quality foods. Eating a handful of almonds instead of snacking on a bag of chips will still satisfy you and help decrease cravings for junk.

Perhaps the bottom line is that many of us equate food with love. The process of eating can have a soothing quality; the act of chewing actually causes the brain to release calming chemicals. We are hardwired to seek out pleasure, and food can serve as one avenue leading to delight or comfort. With awareness, however, we can address the real underlying issues and support ourselves in creating lives we love by making healthier food and, thus, healthier life choices.

Cravings/Food Addictions

Body-Food Relationship coach Anita Avalos hates the term

"food addictions."[14] She points out that using the word "addiction" creates a stressful environment for the eater and contributes to the unhelpful cascade of shame and blame that many people already experience with food. I tend to agree.

That said, I've chosen to employ the term "addiction" here because I think the word "habits" is just not strong enough. While I do want to recognize that the addictive aspect of food can be very real, I use the word "addiction" with caution; I certainly don't want to contribute to creating even more difficulty with the food experience.

Many people view food cravings as *the* toughest roadblock to making healthy choices. A 2008 study[15] regarding the addictive properties of sugar concluded the following: "Food is not ordinarily like a substance of abuse, but intermittent bingeing and deprivation changes that. Based on the observed behavioral and neurochemical similarities between the effects of intermittent sugar access and drugs of abuse, we suggest that sugar, as common as it is, nonetheless meets the criteria for a substance of abuse and may be 'addictive' for some individuals when consumed in a 'binge-like' manner."

Many well-meaning folks fall into dieting practices that create just this sort of dangerous scenario. Meat, cheese and chocolate, as well as some chemical additives and other food substances, also exhibit addictive qualities when consumed repeatedly and in this manner.

While most of us crave sweets and fats (and for good reason: they tend to trigger a release of pleasure chemicals in our brains), keep in mind that we won't be eliminating either in this book. We'll be replacing them with healthy fats (such as avocados, olive oil, nuts and seeds) and natural sugars and fruits, not to mention some really fantastic snacks and desserts, if that's your thing.

Processed food is designed to hit all our pleasure centers at once. As a consequence our taste buds have been over-stimulated and skewed, and the more we eat these foods, the more we *want* to eat them. This is one reason we benefit from the cleansing aspects of the healthy diet—we get to reset our taste buds. Remember biting into a juicy peach or popping a ripe blackberry into your mouth as a kid? Junk food dumbs down our ability to actually taste our food. When we reset, we find out what our bodies truly need underneath the overstimulation. Then we get to experience the deliciousness of foods the way nature made them.

While cravings can indicate that something is missing from an individual's lifestyle or diet, keep in mind that if the body is used to receiving junk food, it will typically continue to crave it until it detoxes out. Even if we downplay the addictive quality of certain foods, the familiarity factor still comes into play. Remember, we tend to reach for what we're used to.

On top of all that, if your body's GPS is clogged by toxins, unfamiliar chemicals and inflammation-producing foods, it can't tell you what it needs with the clarity required. It's just too busy putting out fires and dealing with the onslaught of junk. Additionally, if we're not used to tuning in to our bodies, we may not hear the cues, even if our bodies are screaming at us.

As a society, we've grown accustomed to numbing out and ignoring our bodies in every way except aesthetically. Have pain? Take a painkiller! Skin looks wan? Cover it with makeup! For most of us, our bodies are trying to catch up with what may be a massive clean-up job due to the unhealthy substances we ingest. Like the environment, if we don't turn things around, our bodies may eventually lose the battle and begin to shut down.

With that said, here are some ideas to address food cravings:

- Availability: simply make those unhealthy, craved foods unavailable. Throw them away and don't allow them back into your space. Avoid walking down tempting aisles in the grocery store and just drive on by fast food havens. Enlist the help of family members in creating a healthy eating zone in your home. Granted, this can be difficult when cohabitating with other folks used to eating unhealthily. In that case, share your reasons for improving your eating habits and general health with your family or roommates—not to convince them to do the same, but simply to ask for their support on your own journey.

- Talk about it: hiding creates shame and increases resistance. If and when you binge, be honest with yourself about it. Talk about it with a trusted friend or coach. Perfection is not going to happen and we shouldn't expect that. We all fall down time and time again; we're human. It's getting back up that counts.

- Shake it up: if you usually drive a particular route home from work and stop at a fast food place for dinner, take a different route. Of course you can't avoid seeing fast food places for the rest of your life, and that's not the point. What we want to do here is break old habits and create new, healthy ones. After a while these places may not even register as you drive by.

- Bring your own food: get in the habit of throwing some easy, healthy snacks in your desk, car, backpack, purse or briefcase. When hunger strikes, it often doesn't matter what makes you full. If you're full, you're full, whether it's on pumpkin seeds or donuts. Make it the easiest thing in the world to choose the pumpkin seeds.

- Substitutes: is there a particular food you crave for which you might find a substitute? What is it about the experience of that particular food that contributes to your desire to eat it? Is it texture? Taste? Location? Association? Do you always eat a salami sandwich at a relative's home or in the park? Try taking sun-dried tomatoes and garlic spread with you instead. Keep trying until you find substitutes you love almost as much as (or more than) the original. You may start craving those instead. I promise this can happen, especially as you get more skilled at making raw foods. Owner and chef Brooke Preston of The Green Boheme in Roseville, California, makes the most amazing bacon—out of zucchini!

- Be patient: Food cravings will start to wane after about two weeks of not giving in to them. It's proven, however, that visual images (either the real thing or photos, such as on a menu) may indeed trigger those cravings again. Recognize that this is what's happening and keep the big picture in mind. Simply say "no" with love.

Now let's look at the theory that cravings may indicate you're missing something in your diet. This can be true (as we addressed in the "Food as Substitution" section), but usually not in a literal sense. Your body will never technically need cheesy puffs or chocolate chip cookies.

If you find yourself craving these kinds of items, however, your body may be signaling for higher fat content or for an emotional need (sweetness or romance perhaps, chocolate lovers?). Some foods tend to cause us to zone out, which can indicate a desire to disconnect from present circumstances. Or they may provide a buzzy, excited feeling that we're missing in our everyday lives. Maybe the food you're craving simply symbolizes comfort.

This is where self-honesty comes in. Get curious and be willing to look at the motivations behind the food. You may be surprised at what you discover! Explore giving yourself what you need with either a healthier food choice or in a real, authentic way in another part of your life.

One more thing: if you find that despite all your efforts and intentions, cravings continue to regularly get the better of you, don't interpret this as failure. *There is no failure here.* There are only consistent steps into wholeness and health. Sometimes that means two steps forward and one step back! Creating lasting habits takes time. If needed, don't hesitate to consult a coach or other professional who specializes in food addictions or other methods of support on your food journey. There's no shame in asking for help. This process is about you returning to vibrant health. Call in as many supports as needed!

Boredom/Lack of Presence

As you begin to observe your eating habits, if you discover that you drift to the fridge when you're bored, stressed or unfocused, you're not alone. Most of us have had the experience of finding that we've eaten an entire bag of chips or cookies without any awareness of having done so. If this is your primary hang-up, you're in luck—it's a relatively simple issue to address. What's more, increasing awareness of the present moment is something that will drastically improve the quality of your life in general. It's also critical in terms of self-honesty, something you'll need in spades for any kind of transition to stick.[16]

Here are some ideas to address this area of resistance:

- Meditation: there's nothing like meditation to experience the present moment. Continued practice leads to ever-expanding consciousness of the here and now and, as an added benefit, greater awareness of what you're consuming.

- Presence practice through food consumption: using meal times to practice being extremely present can eliminate unconscious fridge-raiding and become a beloved practice in BE-ing in the moment.

- Life look: maybe it's time to take a good hard look at how you're spending your time. Are you in a job that doesn't suit you? Too busy? Tolerating a situation that's grown stale? Are you spending enough time moving your body, meeting with friends and expressing yourself? Sometimes boredom and/or lack of presence can signal a desire to disconnect from old patterns that no longer serve you.

- Challenges: is it time to take on some new challenges in your life? Maybe you used to enjoy what you're doing, but it's all become somewhat run-of-the-mill and is no longer a "Hell YES!" for you. Is it time to step up your game, try a new hobby, explore someplace you've never been or learn a new skill? It's possible to step out and try new things just for the fun of it. See if you find renewed passion in an old interest, or new interest in something you've never tried!

Detoxification and Healing

In this chapter we've explored some of the myriad reasons why we eat what we do, and how to begin changing ingrained habits that may have caused us to stumble off the path to well-being. Along the way I mentioned the idea of a "reset."

By reset I mean starting at square one, as free as possible of the toxins, chemicals, allergens and other no-good substances that have infiltrated the Standard American Diet. In the next chapter, we'll be looking a little more closely at some of these ingredients and their impact on your health and that of the planet. For now, I'll just point out that you want to reduce and eventually eliminate them, not only to have a clean and healthy body, but also to clear the airwaves so that when your body talks to you, you'll be able to hear it. The signal will get through without being distorted by interference from a toxic fog, and your intuition will begin to show up in all areas of your life. If you're used to eating in an unhealthy way, or are perhaps allergic to something in your diet, your body is going to need a period of detoxification before it can reset.

The raw food lifestyle can be used as a cleanse. It is, by definition, a very clean way to eat, allowing the body to detoxify and heal naturally on a daily basis. It is also an amazing way to live on a full-time basis.

You may choose to do a couple of days of juicing here and there, a day of water fasting or some other approach as a detox.[17] However, eating raw vegan foods is incredibly cleansing and will, in and of itself, allow your body the rest and detoxification time it needs all on its own. As your body begins to reset itself, it will become far easier for you to listen to and respect what it tells you. Given the chance to detox and reregulate, your body can then become your best friend, ally and personal guide back to health.

NOTE: If you're dealing with a critical health condition, know that, although raw food is often recommended by those in the know for addressing severe issues, as you specifically target your illness and symptoms, there may be extenuating circumstances and considerations in addition to what I present in this book. **Always check with a healthcare provider you trust.**

The body's job is to maintain balance. A varied diet of good quality, organically-grown, whole food provides it the materials to do so efficiently and effectively. I often think it's less about *doing* anything and more about *not* throwing in wrenches and messing up what the human body does naturally. As Dr. Albert Schweitzer once said, "It's supposed to be a secret, but I'll tell you anyway. We doctors do nothing. We only help and encourage the doctor within."

We have all the tools we need to assist in the job: clear out the junk and let the body rest, recover and do its natural job of maintaining balance. Then all we ever have to do is listen for our instructions in the moment.

You Can Do This!

There are many reasons why someone chooses to consume healthy foods, or chooses not to. As we've seen, some of these reasons are highly individualized, but no matter what you find as you begin exploring these questions for yourself, YOU CAN DO THIS!

You may well encounter bumps along the way. At times you

may feel like giving up. That's okay. Just remember that once you're on your way, no packaged cookie or fast food burger will taste as good as how you'll *feel* eating foods that are in alignment with your true self—foods that support functioning at your highest level physically, mentally and emotionally, and which help the planet as well!

It really comes down to three things:

- Prioritizing
- Honoring yourself
- Creating new habits and routines

As we move forward, let's sprinkle in healthy doses of patience, kindness and love every step of the way. As your body gets used to eating healthy foods that make you feel terrific and want to leap out of bed to start your day, *that* will become your motivation.

Chapter Three

What We Won't Be Eating

B efore we begin looking at what we won't be eating, let's briefly remind ourselves of what will be on our plates if we veer away from the Standard American Diet in the health and freedom-expanding direction of raw vegan foods: fruits, vegetables, nuts and seeds.

However, your meals don't have to be of the sticks, berries and birdseed variety! You'll be amazed at the diversity, complexity and deliciousness of raw and living foods, and at how simple they can be to prepare. What's more, if you incline towards the gourmet, you can quickly and easily head in that direction too.

To make room for all this culinary goodness, we'll be removing a few items from our diet. In this chapter we'll talk about the *what* and *why* behind avoiding highly processed and genetically modified foods, toxic chemicals, meat and cooking.

Highly Processed Foods

The term "processed food" refers to foods that have been altered from their natural state in any way. Under that broad definition, we could call sliced veggies processed foods, but that's obviously not what I'm referring to here.

Let's differentiate between highly processed and minimally processed. By minimally processed I mean the slicing, chopping, low-heat (under 118 degrees F°) drying or blending of whole foods. Sometimes freezing can be handy as well. These minimal processes get a pass in my book as they don't alter food enzymes or nutrients to any significant degree.

Chemically altering foods as a type of food processing, however, such as in the hydrogenation of oils, is considered highly processed. This often exacts a price in terms of health. Pasteurization (whether steam or chemical) or the addition of sugars, salt and fats (e.g., trans fats) are other examples of processes that negatively affect food's nutritional value and/or our body's ability to use that food in an optimal manner. One process I often find laughable is "fortifying" foods, as if it's an extra gift, often with ingredients that were removed by another process in the first place!

Typically, highly processed foods are created by a manufacturer to "add value" (extend shelf-life, "improve" flavor or mouth-feel, or alter the food's structure). They also, and not coincidentally I'm afraid, tend to increase the price of the item. None of these extreme processes do anything but degrade the nutritional quality of the food. And they often also interfere with the wonderful flavors available in natural, unprocessed plants.

Foods in their natural state are wondrous works of art, in addition to boasting inherent medicinal qualities and delicious flavors. The more we can stick to eating foods as close to their natural state as possible, the more our bodies will thank us. We co-evolved with plants eaten for sustenance over thousands of years; these plants provide our bodies with information for optimal health. Many processed foods, on the other hand, including those made with added sugar, refined grains or trans fats, have only been mass distributed since the 1950s—not long enough for our systems to know what to do with many of them.

Given this and everything else we've discussed so far, keep this general suggestion in mind: with few exceptions, if it's packaged or highly processed you're better off without it. These kinds of foods are typically laden with substances we want to eliminate for good health.

Just by taking this one step, most people's health will improve dramatically.

Toxic Chemicals

In *The Hundred-Year Lie,* Randall Fitzgerald quotes author Jean Carper, who analyzed and contrasted over 10,000 food studies from the National Library of Medicine in Bethesda, Maryland, and the University of Illinois at Chicago. Based on her analysis, Carper writes:

> Food is the breakthrough drug of the twenty-first century. Despite our man-made wonder drugs, Mother Nature is truly the world's oldest and greatest pharmacist. Mainstream scientists are increasingly reaching back to the truths of ancient food folk medicine and dietary practices.

To this, Fitzgerald adds:

> Foods can induce a range of therapeutic effects on human body functions, acting as anticoagulants, analgesics, sedatives, cholesterol reducers, cancer fighters, immune stimulators, anti-inflammatories and on and on. The medicinal effects of food are synergistic.[18]

Given this knowledge, it's more than a little disturbing that the Standard American Diet is chock full of foods loaded with all sorts of man-made chemicals, residual pesticides, toxins and other questionable substances.

Carper also writes: "A single food contains hundreds or thousands of (natural) chemicals, mostly unidentified, that make up each bite's pharmacological activity."[19]

Is it worth asking what all of our additives are doing to this delicate balance?

Toxic chemicals in our food packaging, food and water are a threat to our health. Let's take a look at some of the chemicals commonly found in our food system.[20]

- PBDEs: chemical flame-retardant residue found in common, name-brand grocery items, including meat and dairy products. These chemicals bioaccumulate (collect in the body) and their long-term effects are still unknown.

- Methyl bromide: a neurotoxic pesticide still used on most crops and golf courses.

- BPA: an endocrine disrupter used in plastic packaging that affects development, memory, intelligence and learning.

- TCP and DDT: mutagenic insecticides affecting reproductive health and detected in 93–99 percent of a random human test sample.

- Teflon: contaminates tap water, which explains why 90 percent of Americans test positive for Teflon in their blood. Linked to birth defects and developmental disorders.

- Perchlorate: rocket fuel (also used in fireworks and auto air bags) which can cause cancer and disrupt thyroid function. Contaminates drinking water for twenty million Americans.

- Chlorine: causes corrosive tissue damage when inhaled. Found in tap water and transformed into gas by showering, humidifiers and dishwashing.

- PPCPs: Pharmaceuticals and Personal Care Products found in municipal sewage that cannot be extracted or filtered out by wastewater treatment plants and which are recycled back into the environment and into tap water. The millions of potential synergistic effects from this deluge have not been (and functionally cannot be) studied.

This is only the tip of the iceberg.

> In the past one hundred years, [reports Randall Fitzgerald in *The Hundred-Year Lie*] our species has been engaged in a vast and complicated chemistry experiment. Each and every one of us, along with our children, our parents, and our grandparents, has been a guinea pig in this experiment, which uses our bodies, our health, our wealth, and our goodwill to test the proposition that modern science can improve upon the foods and medicines of nature.[21]

With the rates of cancer, death from brain diseases such as Alzheimer's and Parkinson's, diabetes and obesity rates (to name a few) increasing, I think it's fair to say the experiment is not going well. Toxicity, Fitzgerald notes, only varies by degree. We are all contaminated, and "with up to one hundred thousand separate synthetic chemicals in production and in the marketplace" at this point, the experiment is clearly out of anyone's control.[22]

Consequently, when we talk about better health now, it's about reduction and detoxification. This takes some conscious effort, but it's certainly possible to accomplish. What we eat is so significant because even though healthy bodies are amazing filters and purifiers, what doesn't get filtered out is often stored in the tissues of the body.

Even if we studiously avoid consuming products and foods containing dangerous chemicals, we still carry a toxic load via the chemicals in our air and water. In spite of this, by taking responsibility for limiting our exposure to these substances and by eating a detoxifying diet we can make a significant difference in our health.

Cleansing our personal environment of as many toxic substances as possible is also key. For example, we can replace chemical cleaning and personal care products in the home with benign products like baking soda and vinegar. Chemical companies don't want you to figure this stuff out, but baking soda can be used as toothpaste, shampoo and household cleaner, among other things. I've personally used it for all these purposes.[23]

In addition, a good air filter will help remove toxins from the air in your home (which is notoriously more toxic than outside air). Installing water filters in your kitchen and shower will provide you with better quality water, and a whole house filter is even better.

These kinds of simple steps, along with making sure your food is of good quality and non-toxic, will ensure you're limiting your exposure to toxins.

In this book, of course, our topic is primarily food, and the surest way to avoid ingesting toxins is to purchase organic foods. Yes, it's often a bit more expensive, but consider this philosophy: spend a little more now and feel great, or pay in doctor's bills and life-quality later. Your choice.

Personally, I just prefer to eat as few known carcinogens and synthetic chemicals as possible.

In the U.S., E.U., Canada, Mexico, Japan and other countries, labeling foods "organic" requires a special certification process. As part of this process, farmers are required to follow certain government regulations when raising their crops.

The United States Department of Agriculture (USDA) organic labeling program also ensures that farms and processors preserve natural resources and biodiversity and support animal health and welfare. This makes sense both in terms of compassion for animals as well as for improving your own health if you do consume meat. According to the USDA, foods labeled as organic must also be "produced without excluded methods (e.g., genetic engineering, ionizing radiation, or sewage sludge)."[24] In general, foods must also not be exposed to prohibited substances, which include synthetic pesticides, poisonous chemicals or chemical mixtures. However, pesticides derived from natural sources are allowed.

Mary Jane Butters, internationally recognized organic farmer, author, environmental activist, and food manufacturer, quips, "I think we need to take back our language. I want to call my organic carrots 'carrots' and let [other farmers] call theirs a 'chemical carrot.' And they can list all of the ingredients that they used instead of me having to be certified."[25]

While I couldn't agree more with Butters' sentiments, as it stands now, things are indeed backwards. Organic labeling is still where it's at when we're looking for the healthiest choices.

Fortunately, due to demand, even many big chain stores are making efforts to provide quality organic food sections. This of course makes buying organic more convenient and cheaper than ever before. My local Ralph's, for example, consistently carries large bunches of fresh, organic kale for ninety-nine cents.

While there are admittedly potential issues with organic farming and its regulation, such as the largely unknown long-term effects of natural pesticides or the negative impacts of the certification process, organic certification is a huge step in the right direction. At the very least, it allows me to be sure I'm not consuming genetically modified organisms, which we'll discuss next.

Genetically Modified Organisms

Genetically modified organisms (GMOs) are foods such as corn and soybeans that have been genetically engineered to, among other things, render them resistant to herbicides and pests or increase their tolerance to environmental conditions such as drought. In the U.S., GM foods include the common crops of papaya, corn, soybeans, zucchini, sugar beets, cotton, canola and others. At this time, nuts and seeds do not contain GMOs.

While many sources purport that scientific studies are not yet showing any negative health impacts on people consuming GMOs, buyer beware. Research on GMOs' impact on human health is quite sparse. Commercial sale of GM crops was initiated in 1994, and new products continue to come to market, so time has yet to tell the whole story. However, as I'll briefly get into in a moment, there do appear to be some grave concerns.

It's worth mentioning, too, that GMOs have not been universally accepted as safe by the scientific and medical communities. The American Academy of Environmental Medicine, for example, offers a Position Statement on GMOs that reads in part, "There is more than a casual association between GM foods and adverse health effects. There is causation as defined by Hill's Criteria in the areas of strength of association, consistency, specificity, biological gradient, and biological plausibility. The strength of association and consistency between GM foods and disease is confirmed in several animal studies." The group further calls for "a moratorium on GM food, implementation of immediate long term independent safety testing, and labeling of GM foods, which is necessary for the health and safety of consumers."[26]

More than sixty GM crops have been approved for U.S. food and feed supplies and new ones are approved each year. Livestock feed is also usually manufactured using GM crops. As I write this, sixty-four countries require GM labeling.[27] Polls indicate that over 90% of Americans are in favor of labeling.[28] Thankfully, in May of 2018 the USDA released a draft ruling calling for foods containing GMOs to be labeled as "bioengineered," or "BE." This rule went into effect on January 1, 2020, with a mandatory compliance date of January 1, 2022.[29] While this is definitely a step in the right direction, critics of the labeling program point out that the rule has several problems that make it far from perfect. For example, it "does not clearly require the disclosure of all genetically engineered ingredients, including highly refined sugars and oils, and new GM techniques like CRISPR and RNAi."[30]

Under the pressure of consumer outcry, and after spending billions to keep consumers in the dark about GM ingredients, several large companies including ConAgra, Mars, General Mills and Campbell's are seeing the writing on the wall and are pledging to voluntarily label their products.

Over 70 percent of packaged foods sold in the U.S. contain GMOs.[31] So even if we are not directly eating the whole GM food (such as may be the case with soybeans or corn), GMOs are included as all kinds of additives in packaged foods. The only sure way to eliminate GMOs from your diet is to buy organic or check for labeling which ensures that the product has been independently third-party verified GMO-free by an organization such as the Non-GMO Project.

Conventional agriculture has also modified food via cross-breeding and hybridization with existing species of similar organisms, such as with different strains of corn. Modern genetic engineering techniques, however, can actually splice genes of different species into one organism (as is the case, for example, with corn modified to include the bacteria *Bacillus thuringiensis*, or Bt).

While conventional cross-breeding and hybridization do not pose health threats, the same may not be true for GMOs. Because of the difficulties involved in isolating particular chemicals in food, GM foods do not undergo the types of human testing that, for example, a new drug typically undergoes before being released to the market. Rather, they are usually considered to be "substantially equivalent" to their non-GMO counterparts and are therefore not required to undergo rigorous safety testing.[32]

Some studies are finding evidence that GMO foods may not be all they're cracked up to be. For example, a 2006 study from the Danish Institute for Food and Veterinary Research found that the Bt toxin, a biological pesticide incorporated into the DNA of certain crops, can remain in the gut after being ingested.[33] Bt works to kill insects, such as beetles, caterpillars and butterflies, by paralyzing their digestive systems so that they stop eating and starve to death.[34] Researchers found that when foods genetically modified to produce their own Bt toxin are eaten, the toxin continues to be produced in the gut. The long-term effects of this are uncertain.

Other research is underway regarding the herbicide glyphosate, first developed by Monsanto in the 1970s and used extensively on GM crops and throughout the agricultural system in the U.S.[35,36] Glyphosate is a broad-spectrum, nonselective systemic herbicide; it doesn't simply act on one particular type of plant, but on *all* plants. Among other troubling effects on human systems, glyphosate may act as an antibiotic when introduced into the human body, causing gut dysbiosis by killing beneficial organisms while allowing pathogenic organisms to proliferate. It is also potentially implicated in multiple conditions such as autism, liver necrosis, infertility and birth defects.[37,38]

Additional big-picture complications with GMO crops include:

- The evolution of pesticide/herbicide resistant "superweeds" and "superbugs". In a never-ending cycle to eradicate these new offenders, more and stronger toxins are being applied, resulting in increased negative health effects for humans, animals and the environment[39] without proof that crops are of higher quality or more prolific.

- The concern that GMO crops inspire an even greater reliance on monoculture, a farming practice that can devastate species and seed diversity.[40]

- The monstrous concern of corporate control which transfers seed ownership from farmers to industrial giants (most notably Monsanto). These chemical companies acquire seed patents and sue farmers for patent infringement when their fields become contaminated by GM pollen or seeds. This results in massive disruption, loss of livelihood and market destruction, particularly in developing nations where 70 percent of the populations support their households with food production.[41]

In any case, the experiment is ongoing. If you eat GMO foods, know that you and your children (whose systems are less tolerant than an adult's) are the guinea pigs. This is a very complex topic, and not one that we can explore in great depth here. But interested readers are encouraged to do their own research and to stay informed about the latest products released to market and the current state of the scientific research.

Animals and Animal Products

Eliminating the consumption of animals and animal products will also be key to optimal health for us and the planet. Why?

First of all, nutritional research points hands-down to a balanced, whole foods, plant-based diet as the healthiest way to eat.[42]

In 2015 the World Health Organization convened a panel of twenty-two experts from ten different countries to review over eight hundred studies and concluded that eating processed meat such as hot dogs or bacon raises the risk of colon cancer.[43] They also noted that consuming other red meats most likely raises the risk of cancer as well.

Decades ago, studies indicating dire health impacts caused by meat consumption were deliberately withheld from the public. The McGovern Committee released their report *Dietary Goals for the United States* in 1977, which recommended decreasing consumption of animal-based foods and increasing intake of plant-based foods. Not surprisingly, this report was met with strong push-back from the meat and dairy industries, and amid a dramatic bureaucratic melee, the report was eventually suppressed.[44]

Some additional data follows.

In his 2013 lecture "Uprooting the Causes of Death,"[45] Dr. Michael Greger reviews the literature and concludes that eating a vegan diet drastically reduces the risk of dying from almost all of the top killers in the United States, including heart disease, diabetes and stroke.

Research by biochemist T. Colin Campbell and physician

Thomas M. Campbell demonstrates that "there are virtually no nutrients in animal-based foods that are not better provided by plants."[46] Their work, published in *The China Study,* draws on the results of a massive, twenty-year project providing a plethora of scientific data in support of a plant-based diet. [47]

For the planet, meat consumption is simply not a sustainable practice in the long run.[48] Eliminating meat not only decreases the incidence of animal suffering, but is also critical for the health of the environment. While this topic could fill an entire book in itself, here are a few of the ways that eating vegan positively impacts the Earth and everyone on it. Switching to a plant-based diet:

- Reduces water consumption. In general, fruits and veggies require significantly less water to produce than meat. While global figures vary, it takes between 2,500– 5,000 gallons of water to produce one pound of beef, as opposed to fifteen gallons to produce a pound of lettuce, or fifty-five gallons for oranges.

- Eliminates/drastically reduces packaging waste. With the current pollution issue, including the great Pacific garbage patch,[49] anything we can do to reduce or eliminate the use of plastics in our lives is a very good thing. Raw, fresh fruits and vegetables come in their own containers! While some stores are guilty of over-packaging their produce, you can avoid the plastic trap by purchasing from the bulk section and from sources that use minimal packing or eliminate it altogether. Bringing your own reusable bags is key as well. With the exception of small individual fruits like grape tomatoes and raspberries, even my local Ralph's does not generally package their produce. Farmers' markets are another sure bet.

- Saves fossil fuels. One third of all fossil fuels consumed in the U.S. are used in animal production. As a comparison, fifty-four calories of fossil fuels are needed for production of one calorie of protein from beef, while only three calories of fossil fuels are required to produce one calorie of protein from corn.[50]

- Frees up land use. Livestock consumes the majority of the world's crops. In fact, 40 percent of our planet's land surface is used by livestock or for growing food for those animals. According to Jonathan Foley, Heinz Award recipient from the University of Minnesota's Institute on the Environment, that's sixty times more area than our cities and suburbs take up.[51]

- Decreases deforestation and desertification. It's been known for some time that rainforests in Brazil are being razed for livestock grazing and feed use, yet rainforest destruction continues to be a significant issue across the planet. Currently the vast majority of global land-use issues originate in the agricultural sector, primarily driven by the demand for space for cattle, other livestock and feed crops.

- Decreases pollution. The pollution issue is an enormous one, and raising livestock is a massive contributor to this problem. Livestock, for instance, is one of the main sources of the world's methane emissions. Greenhouse gasses are also generated during livestock "production" in terms of animal waste management.[52] Antibiotics, nutrients, heavy metals, growth hormones and other chemicals that Concentrated Animal Feeding Operations (CAFOs) introduce into the environment are also major pollutants. Another fact: 37 percent of pesticide use is concentrated on animal feed crops alone.

- Decreases incidence of starvation. Because meat requires more resources to produce, it is less efficient at feeding large numbers of people than a plant-based diet. Consider the following from an article published in *Earthoria*: "There is more than enough food in the world to feed the entire human population. So why are more than 840 million people still going hungry? . . . The more meat we eat, the fewer people we can feed. If everyone on Earth received 25 percent of his or her calories from animal products, only 3.2 billion people would have food to eat. Dropping that figure to 15 percent would mean that 4.2 billion people could be fed. If the whole world became vegan, there would be plenty of food to feed all of us." [53] That's more than 7.7 billion people. The Worldwatch Institute sums this up, saying, "Meat consumption is an inefficient use of grain . . . Grain is used more efficiently when consumed by humans. Continued growth in meat output is dependent on feeding grain to animals, creating competition for grain between affluent meat-eaters and the world's poor."[54]

- Eliminates/drastically reduces animal suffering. Even in the best of situations, meat consumption requires the death of fellow creatures—creatures who instinctively want to live, to enjoy the sun and the sky and the grass as much as you or I. The fact is that *all* creatures, even an amoeba, will attempt to evade death. In the worst of situations (of which many still exist today), animals live short lives filled with suffering, depression, terrible living conditions, cruelty and pain. CAFOs not only pollute the environment but also carry out the raising and slaughtering of animals as "products," irrespective of any honor or care for the conscious creatures that are their victims.

Heat Processing

Okay, vegan is obviously great for us and for the planet. Why, then, would we go further and make the leap from vegan to *raw* vegan? Several reasons.

First are the biochemical ones. A raw vegan diet is rich in intact nutrients. Raw foods almost always contain more fiber, vitamins, minerals, protein, antioxidants and phytochemicals than their cooked counterparts. Most foods are more nutritious when eaten raw, as cooking degrades or destroys many vital nutrients. Much of the cooked food we eat can also be highly processed, full of saturated fats, trans fats, excess sodium and so on. (Fortunately at this point, 98 percent of trans-fats have been removed from the food system as the result of a recent ban enacted June 18, 2019.) As we've discussed already, eliminating these from our diet can do wonders for our health.

Furthermore, cooking often denatures proteins, meaning it alters their natural structure and can affect the way they are absorbed (or not absorbed) by the body. The question posed to many raw vegans, "Where do you get your protein?" is a common one. Many people don't realize that cooking destroys around 50 percent of proteins, and that a varied, raw, plant-based diet contains the exact amount of protein recommended for human consumption (right around 10 percent). Green leafy vegetables contain the highest amount of protein in a raw vegan diet.

Animal food obviously does contain protein (which, incidentally, is derived from plant consumption). However, this protein is not in a form that is available for absorption by humans. The body must break down animal proteins into their separate parts (amino acids) and reformulate these amino acids into chains (proteins) available for human use. This takes energy, and it is much more efficient for the body to create its own usable proteins from the amino acids found in plants. By not cooking plants, amino acids are not destroyed and proteins can easily be assembled and assimilated by the human body.

Cooking also creates chemical compounds that include carcinogens and genotoxic substances, which cause damage at the DNA level.

Many raw foodists also cite living enzymes as a plus for consuming only raw foods. This is based on the idea that enzymes in food typically aid in digestion and other beneficial chemical reactions in the body. Cooking typically destroys these enzymes.

According to some sources, this issue is still up for debate. Some evidence suggests that enzymes are denatured when they contact stomach acid anyway, and that plant enzymes do not actually catalyze chemical reactions for human digestion. However, others claim that enzymes are only inactivated by stomach acid, and they reactivate again in the small intestine.

So while the jury's still out on enzymes, I hope that at this point you have a better appreciation of how a raw vegan diet can help you *and* the planet. We've covered a lot of ground here, and of course there's more to be covered, given the vast amount of research done on the topic. If you're interested in pursuing it further I've provided a preliminary list of books, research studies, TED Talks, blogs and other resources at the end of this book.

For now I'll sum it up in this way: There are many personal and planetary benefits to eating an organic, raw, plant-based diet. I have not, in fact, found any credible arguments against doing so. But if you haven't experienced a raw vegan diet for yourself, it's still all just academic.

Now it's time to see if raw will work for *you*.

Chapter Four

Raw: Is It for You?

So we've reached a decision point. Are you inspired to try eating more raw food?

You've heard many of the pros: besides improving overall health, a raw vegan diet can play a supportive, catalytic role in other areas of your life as well as helping the planet. Healthy weight maintenance, spiritual clarity and improved mental functioning are a few of the life-changing benefits of a raw food diet.

Put simply, eating raw vegan boasts undeniable and massive benefits. Perhaps most importantly, this way of eating can return you to a state of healthy connection with your body and true self.

If you decide to go raw, understand that there will probably be growing pains in terms of the time you spend educating yourself, investing in new equipment and learning new ways to prepare food, but this is true for almost any significant new endeavor. I encourage you to give it a trial period first and see what happens. The only way you'll know how your body responds to this way of eating and whether it will fit into your life is to give it a fair shot. Alternatively, simply adding more raw foods into your current diet will do nothing but benefit you.

Are You In?

If so, terrific! Welcome aboard! Welcome to a life in which you may just feel the best you've ever felt, mentally and physically. Where the need for most medications disappears. Where you find yourself awake and alert, looking yourself and life squarely in the eye. Good for you! Let me repeat: Please allow yourself an unlimited amount of love and patience during your transition.

Also, *please check with your doctor before you begin this or any new regimen*, and of course consult with your physician if you run into any health issues along the way.

And another thing I should mention:

> ♥ *Listen to your body, listen to your body,*
> *listen to your body!* ♥

Your own experiences and feelings will be your best guides moving forward—you'll most likely find that you do well on some raw foods and not on others. Use this book as a blueprint, but also use your own best judgment and strive to eat the most varied, organic, balanced diet you can. Consult additional resources (including naturopathic physicians, supportive and knowledgeable nutritionists and other health professionals), especially if you find yourself feeling less than awesome.

Are you ready?

Fantastic.

Let's get down to the nuts and bolts of this thing!

Part II

How to Go Raw:
The Nuts & Bolts

Chapter Five

The Kitchen

The right equipment will facilitate your transition to the raw food lifestyle. Let's look at some of the tools of the trade.

Kitchen Equipment: Your Healing Tools

Can you sustain a raw food lifestyle with just a knife and cutting board? While others might say "yes," I disagree. You might be able to keep it going for a few days or even weeks, but in my opinion you'll need some special gear to create a variety of nutritious, good-tasting raw foods that you'll enjoy eating on a long-term basis.

Every kitchen requires equipment; the raw food kitchen simply features different equipment. Instead of the standard stove, oven, toaster, coffee maker and pots and pans, the raw food kitchen may boast a high-powered blender, food processor, juicer, spiralizer, and dehydrator. You'll still give that cutting board lots of mileage, too.

Don't worry: you don't need to rush out and acquire all these tools at once, and if you can find used items in good shape, go right ahead. I've spotted decent juicers at thrift stores, and I have a friend who picked up a high-powered blender at a garage sale. Scouring online local-items-for-sale apps and sites can yield some real gems as well. Plow through a local restaurant supply store that carries used items and you'll likely find a variety of fascinating tools and appliances. At the very least you can purchase some great used knives and other hand tools for next to nothing.

If you're just starting out and aren't sure the raw food lifestyle is for you, consider borrowing appliances whenever possible. You might even think about buying less expensive versions to test the waters, if that makes sense with your personal budget. Keep in mind, though, that higher quality equipment (particularly blenders) will often result in preferable food quality.

If, on the other hand, you're positive that raw food is your path, then by all means invest in machines that will serve you for many years to come. With good care and maintenance, I expect my own appliances to last my lifetime. I purchased each piece of equipment one at a time. You can do the same or go all out and buy everything at once.

In deciding what, if any, equipment you may want to buy first, I suggest focusing on filtered water, green smoothies and green juices to start. Just taking these first steps is likely to rapidly do wonders for your health and motivate you to continue to explore. This means looking at water filters, blenders, and juicers. Specific tips and tricks for each item will be provided further on.

Appliances

- Water filter
- High-speed blender
- Food processor
- Juicer
- Dehydrator
- Spiralizer (cuts veggies into noodles)

You'll also need a pretty good-sized fridge, but other than that, you're good to go!

Supplemental Items

Here are some smaller items you might find nice to have around. (I consider the starred items essential.) You probably own most of these already.

- ★ A couple of excellent knives
- ★ Cutting boards (wood is best; it self-heals, is naturally more hygienic and you're not eating plastic particles)
- ★ Citrus juicer (an old-fashioned glass hand-juicer will do)
- ★ Jars for storing nuts and seeds (any variety of wide-mouth jar will work—my favorites are recycled sauerkraut and coconut oil jars)
- ★ Containers and lids for soaking nuts and seeds (large measuring cups or salad/mixing bowls are perfect)
- ★ Mesh nut mylk bags or mesh produce bags for nut mylk and seed-sprouting
- ★ Sports bottles with wide mouths for smoothies and juices (I like the ones made by BlenderBottle)
- ★ Brush for cleaning juicer and spiralizer (a toothbrush will do the job)
- ★ Electric tea kettle for warming tea and cereal, and for sterilization purposes
- • Apple corer/slicer
- • Rubber and angled spatulas (for smoothing items on dehydrator sheets)
- • Mandoline slicer
- • Grater

- Measuring cups and spoons

- Mesh colander

- Coco Jack (very handy for opening coconuts and removing the meat)

- Various hand tools, including a pie server, ladle, ice-cream scooper, salad tongs and large spoons

Appliance-Specific Tips

Let's take a look at each of the larger pieces of equipment in turn.

Water Filter

First of all, why filter tap water at all? Isn't it already safe? In a word, no.

Tap water is generally contaminated with numerous chemicals, including arsenic, pesticides and chlorine. In 2019, the Environmental Working Group found multiple contaminants in U.S. drinking water, many of which aren't regulated by the EPA.[55] Chlorine itself is a suspected carcinogen.

Given our goal of overall health, keeping our internal systems as free of chemicals as possible makes a water filter an important purchase. A filter can remove or at least reduce these contaminants.

While a whole house filter is divine, even water filter pitchers will be a giant boon. Pitchers are readily available and easily maintained by periodically replacing the filters. You can compare brands by doing an Internet search. Under-the-counter, whole-house and faucet filters can also be obtained at a significantly higher cost, and filters run from very affordable to super expensive. While generally you get what you pay for here, with all of these items, even purchasing the cheapest models will be an overall improvement, and you can upgrade along the way if you'd like. I have used Aquasana filters for many years, although I recently switched to a whole-house filter and there is nothing like it!

Whichever filtering system you choose, I also suggest purchasing a filtering water bottle as well. It's great for everyday use and eliminates traditional bottled water waste. When traveling I use it for drinking as well as for washing my face (my skin hates chlorine).

I also suggest using a shower filter; we breathe in contaminants such as chlorine gas emitted in shower spray and also absorb them through our skin.

High-speed Blender

You'll be using your blender almost daily. While other raw foodists may suggest simply using your regular blender when going raw, in the long run you will most likely find this approach unsatisfactory. If the texture of your food means anything to you, think twice about relying on a lower-end blender for too long.

Why? *Mystery chunks.* Using a regular blender often leaves you with chunky globs of you're-often-not-sure-what. Even if you know exactly what's in those chunks they can still be less than appetizing. One of my least favorite snacks early on was a green smoothie straight out of my old $29.99 grocery store blender: lumpy, leafy, sandy and just plain gross. I couldn't handle it, and I still can't!

Moreover, there's no way to create thoroughly blended soups, pulverize seeds or make flour with an inferior blender. And just try to blend nuts into a smooth sauce—good luck! A high-powered blender will also allow you to warm soups. In my opinion, as soon as you can afford a top-of-the-line blender, such as a Vitamix or Blendtec (Vitamix is my favorite), get one. Spend your big money here and thank yourself later; your blender will become a most important raw food ally.

Food Processor

You'll constantly use this tool to create everything from ice cream to taco "meat." The good news is that a raw chef friend of mine suggests picking up the cheapest model possible. He doesn't see any significant difference between a $30 food processor and the $300 machines they use at his restaurant. But *do* get a large one! Mine holds fourteen cups and is large enough for almost everything I do. You can't imagine how tedious it is to make four batches of the same thing when you could have done it all in one fell swoop. I've spent weekends at friends' homes fiddling around with a smaller-sized processor and it's a royal pain in the neck. If your vision is to make your raw food lifestyle sustainable, do yourself a favor and go with a large-sized processor.

Juicer

Like your blender, a juicer is probably one of the more expensive items you'll purchase, but also one of the most important.

Juicing in the mornings changed my health completely. The vitamins and minerals absorbed via a morning vegetable juice are priceless. And it tastes so good! I started out with a Breville Juice Fountain Elite (priced around $300), which I loved, and I've also purchased a Black & Decker (basically a plastic copy of the Breville) for $50; I'm fairly happy with that as well. I have used the Black & Decker for travel and as a backup juicer and have also happily used a Jack LaLanne model. I then moved to the Omega NC800 as my main juicer. You can also use this model to make nut butter and ice cream, and I've been over-the-moon happy with its performance, particularly with leafy greens. Recently, however, I've gone back to the Breville, as with a new baby in the mix, I'm cutting corners where I can to save time, and the Breville requires less prep than the smaller mouthed Omega. More on juicer pros and cons coming up.

Juicers come in several basic types: two-step triturator/hydraulic press, twin gear, masticating, centrifugal basket, and centrifugal pulp-ejecting. You don't need to memorize all that. Juicers are an entire industry in themselves. If you want to research, for example, enzymatic activity as related to juicer types, a good place to start might be with Michael Donaldson, Ph.D.,[56] who provided the above breakdown of juicer types. Donaldson noted that the two-step triturator/hydraulic press resulted in the highest enzymatic activity, while centrifugal juicers had the lowest. Ease of use stats, however, were flipped, with the centrifugal juicer being the simplest to operate and the two-step the most difficult.

While you can go hog wild and spend upwards of $2500 for a Norwalk press juicer, you can also purchase relatively inexpensive juicers of each type. If you're ready, make an investment in a juicer that will last for years. I'll keep things simple here. The pros and cons discussion below will stick to the two main types of juicers (and the ones with which I'm most familiar), which are also the most common and easily operated machines: centrifugal and masticating.

Centrifugal Juicer

Juice is separated from the pulp by a spinning metal blade and filtered through a wire mesh basket-type filter.

Pros

- Fast.
- Simple to use.
- Large intake opening (reduces prep time).

Cons

- Generates some heat while running. While there is debate about the impact of heat on the nutritional content of juice, it is generally felt that the higher the temperature to which juice is heated, the greater the oxidation and destruction of nutrients. Heating also decreases the amount of time juice may be stored (normally it can be stored for up to twenty-four hours with a centrifugal juicer; however, oxidation begins immediately, and the sooner you drink it the better).

- Somewhat less efficient than other types of juicers. Does not extract as much juice from vegetables in general, and from green leafy vegetables in particular.

- Noisy.

Masticating Juicer

The masticating juicer crushes or presses produce to separate the pulp from the juice.

Pros

- Nutrients remain generally intact.

- Little to no heat produced during operation, which translates into less oxidation and longer-lasting juice (can be stored 48–72 hours, depending on the juicer).

- Efficient with greens as well as bulkier items.

- Can be used to make ice creams, nut mylks and butters as well.

- Quieter.

Cons

- Juice extraction tends to be a bit slower with this type of juicer.

- The intake is significantly smaller than most centrifugals, resulting in increased prep time (cutting veggies to fit through the mouth).

- Price can exceed that of centrifugal juicers.

Which juicer should you purchase? This is a call based on your lifestyle, health goals, budget and personal preferences. However, the important thing is to simply *get* a juicer.

No wait—I take that back. The *most* important thing is to *use* your juicer once you have it!

Dehydrator

I ate fully raw for about a year before I finally purchased a dehydrator. But when I did, wow, was I glad!

A dehydrator adds a lot of versatility to your diet. I generally run my dehydrator about four days a week, making treats such as tortillas, naan bread, cookies, burgers, falafel, pizza, bread and protein bars. I also use it for dehydrating the nuts and seeds I soak and sprout, which makes them taste great and allows me to store them for months longer than if they were simply soaked (soaked fridge life spans only a few days).

If you purchase a dehydrator, it needs to have a temperature control. Anything heated over 118 degrees is no longer raw; you might as well use your oven. Some people *do* use their ovens to dehydrate by adjusting the heating to the lowest heat setting and keeping the door ajar. The disadvantage of this approach is that you can't truly control the temperature and may overheat your items, defeating the whole purpose of eating raw.

The Excalibur is an excellent quality dehydrator with a temperature control and timer (on the newer models). The fan is also located at the back of the unit, creating an evenly dehydrated product. If you do choose to purchase this dehydrator, go with a nine-tray. Even when I was only making food for myself I was so happy I had the bigger size. When making items with any height (cookies, bread or kale chips, etc.), you'll need to remove alternating trays to fit everything in (some dehydrators do not allow this flexibility). Suddenly, you have a four-tray dehydrator! If you prepare anything really large (my favorite is a calzone), you'll need to remove several trays at a time.

Go big or go home on this one too!

Spiralizer

While you don't absolutely need this little gem, you can pick one up for around $25–$30 and it's a great tool to keep in your raw tool chest. It's very simple to use and clean, and it allows you to transform cucumbers, beets, zucchini and summer squash (or whatever you're brave enough to try) into noodles, which adds fun and variety to your meals. These veggie noodles are a really nice and quick menu option. Just whip up some easy sauce and in ten minutes you've created a nutritious, delicious meal. I recommend purchasing the larger model with a handle, not the hand-held version, which I found annoyingly slow to use but could be great for travel.

Cleaning Your Appliances

A quick note about cleaning your appliances: I've heard from many people that they don't like to use their juicers (or even blenders) because they don't want to clean them. I get that, and I used to feel the same way.

If this is you, I encourage you to recreate a little experiment I did for myself: set the stopwatch on your phone and time how long it actually takes you to clean your appliance. What I found was that it took me two to three minutes to clean my juicer, and my blender takes even less time than that! In my opinion, your health is certainly worth these couple of minutes per day.

General Kitchen Tips

I've come up with these systems, ideas and tips over the years and have found them incredibly useful. I mention some of these throughout the food section as well, as reminders.

Storage

- Store your dehydrated nuts and seeds in glass jars in fridge doors or in a separate cabinet; it's easy to see what you've got. I use old sauerkraut or coconut oil jars with wide mouths that are easy to pour food into and to clean.

- Create separate storage areas in your fridge for your juice and smoothie items. I have used metal baskets or restaurant storage containers (my favorite, and they can be purchased at restaurant supply stores). That way when you want to make a juice or smoothie, you simply pull out the container and everything you need is at your fingertips. I also have a basket I use for berries and one for vitamins/supplements. An organized fridge will make your raw vegan life much easier.

- Store refrigerated veggies in bags made from flour sack towels. Wet the bag prior to inserting veggies and keep a small spray bottle of water in the fridge door to re-moisten as needed. Veggies stay fresh for a long time using this method.

- Invest in quite a few lidded glass storage containers. Pyrex is a good bet. You don't want to use plastic (even BPA-free plastic is not without its concerns), and you'll use these often to store your yummy leftovers.

- Use your oven for storage! Since I don't use my oven for cooking, over the years I've used it to store my dish linens, protein powders and dishes, and as the perfect-height stand up desk!

- I've also placed an old butcher block-like table top over the top of the cooktop, which serves as an extra countertop and houses my dehydrator, blender, food processor and juicer. My spice rack stands on the back of the stove.

Juicing

- Juicing system: Pull out a small cutting board, knife and tray to hold the cut-up veggies that are ready to go (a metal baking tray with shallow sides is perfect and won't allow water to escape). If possible, place them all near the sink or in an easily accessible drawer. Take out your juicer basket, put it on the counter next to the sink and begin to wash and cut up veggies, placing them on the tray as you go. When ready to juice, place your hand on your tray of veggies, close your eyes and feel your gratitude for and connection to all of this delicious, nutritious, life-giving food! Now, juice!

- I sometimes strain my green juice before drinking it; I prefer the pulp-less texture. I use a fairly large strainer set over a large measuring bowl prior to pouring the juice into a drinking glass or container, using the stirring action of a spoon to force the juice through the strainer as I go.

- Invest in a collection of Blender Bottles (or your favorite lidded sports-drink bottle that's easy to clean) for smoothies and juices. For years I got by with two of these and finally invested in quite a few more—I can't believe it took me so long! I use these daily and usually have at least four in the fridge with smoothies and juices ready to go. They're terrific for travel and taking to work. I keep mine corralled in a repurposed wire container in my cupboard where they're easily accessible, with their corresponding lids in a container next to them.

Miscellaneous

- Keep a cardboard box lined with a large plastic bag in the freezer. Throw any compostable food scraps in there and save yourself a) a stinky outside trash can and b) running out to dump the scraps all the time. The frozen scraps will not stick to the plastic bag, so reuse the bag every time. Most of your kitchen waste will be food scraps, and this works amazingly. Dump it once a week in the green waste on trash day, if your area has such a program in place.

- Always use nut mylk bags with the seams turned outward. This makes them much easier to clean, which you can do at the sink with a little dish soap and elbow grease.

- Keep a trio of insulated lunch bags at the ready. I have a larger one for day trips and flights, one that's the perfect size for two Blender Bottles filled with juice and/or smoothie (and an ice sheet), and one for my regular lunch. I rarely leave home for any period of time without one of the three next to me in the car.

- Pour dehydrated nuts and seeds into jars by lifting the Teflex and/or base screen off of the dehydrator shelf, pulling the sides together and making a "slide."

- Turn dehydrated items by removing the item's tray, removing another empty tray and placing it over the items (making a tray "sandwich") and then turning both trays before removing the original one.

- Keep a variety of ice sheets and packs in your freezer at all times.

- Cleaning products: the only home cleaning products I use are baking soda, vinegar, Dr. Bronner's liquid soap, and water. You can add essential oils if you're big on aromas—they can be very nice and add their own antiseptic (and healing) properties. White vinegar is a terrific disinfectant, deodorizer and degreaser. Additionally, it kills eensy-weensies we'd rather not have around such as Salmonella, E. coli and other Gram-negative bacteria—all while being completely non-toxic to us. You don't want to add to indoor air pollution by using chemical products, and really, you don't need them. I highly recommend Karyn Siegel-Maier's useful little volume *The Naturally Clean Home* for nontoxic cleaning formulas.

♥   ♥   ♥

That's it! Raw food preparation can be as simple as biting into an apple or as complex as creating a multi-layer, exquisitely delicious dessert. With the appropriate tools and equipment on hand, you can expand your raw food repertoire as you become more familiar with ingredients and techniques and dive further into the adventure of the raw food experience.

Chapter Six

Meals and Meal Plans

One of the first questions I'm asked by people who are curious about how I eat is,

"But aren't you hungry all the time??"

NO! I only eat when I'm hungry, which, if you're wondering, is *not* all the time! I'm not into self-deprivation, and if I felt hungry all the time I'd certainly change my eating habits. I eat until I'm full and then I eat again when I'm hungry. My body is completely competent at self-regulation.

The second question I'm repeatedly asked is, "But what do you actually *eat??*" I'm about to answer that.

The Structured Plan

I'm not one for prescribed anything, let alone prescribed *eating*. However . . .

Over the years, I've developed a loose structure that makes eating quite simple and requires very little thought or planning. Many raw food experts actually suggest planning your meals this way; however, my body just prefers simplicity and came to this "plan" on its own. I'm going to provide you with this overall structure, which is ultimately customizable to your own needs and preferences. You can vary the content with the seasons and your own preferences, moving within the structure while knowing you're consuming many different foods to keep you healthy—without being bored to tears in the process.

Here's the structured plan, along with my daily wellness routine:

Morning

- Upon waking (typically between 5:00 and 7:00 a.m.): large glass of filtered water with lemon juice or a tablespoon or two of apple cider vinegar (I also drink filtered water throughout the day and with each meal). After this I walk my dog and get a little nature connection time in.

- Half an hour or so later: 8 ounces-ish of homemade kombucha and a pinch of miso or a few bites of sauerkraut (probiotic foods are great for promoting heathy gut flora). I periodically add a probiotic supplement here as well—give this step at least half an hour before you introduce juice or other food. Those probiotics benefit from a little alone-time to properly make themselves at home!

- Half an hour or so later: large glass of fresh green juice (I often make my juice a little while after finishing my kombucha and then drink the juice directly after I make it—generally I prepare two juices and refrigerate one for the next day) followed by light yoga stretching and meditation.

- Breakfast: cereal, chia seeds, fruit (half a cantaloupe with cinnamon is fantastic in the summer!), nut bar or green smoothie (usually a smoothie—here again, I typically prepare two smoothies and refrigerate one for the evening or for the next day). Then I get to work on my projects for the day.

- Snack: fruit, nuts, seeds or veggies.

Afternoon

- Lunch: my heaviest meal of the day. Typically, a nut or seed pâté in or on a veggie or wrap/tortilla (e.g., tostada), avocado, hummus, a burger, soup, or pasta with sauce, etc. I may enjoy a piece of fruit as well and often head to the gym for an hour or so.

Evening

- Dinner (I do my best to eat before 7:00 p.m., before my evening dog walk and meditation): typically I drink another green smoothie or juice, enjoy a large salad or finish up lunch leftovers.

- Dessert: I very rarely eat dessert; I don't have much of a sweet tooth. However, sometimes I'm in the mood and I'll eat a date or a macaroon or make an easy dessert, such as banana ice-cream, apple pie, or berries with nut cream. I will also sometimes eat these as a snack in the middle of the day.

- I like to use only candlelight at night (and no screens after dark; the blue light emitted negatively impacts melatonin production and significantly disrupts sleep cycles). I'm typically in bed snoozing by 9:00 or 10:00 p.m.

Within this structure, I feel great and have all the freedom in the world. I make use of loads of fresh local fruit in the summers and enjoy trying new recipes, often raw renditions of ethnic foods I love. The main ingredients are almost always *ease* and *simplicity*.

Mixing It Up

Here are some ideas for mixing things up within your meal plan:

- Rotate in different varieties of nuts and seeds. There are a ton of them out there, and they all feature different important nutrients.

- Use seasonal produce. A Community Supported Agriculture (CSA) box is perfect for this, and so convenient! Using seasonal produce automatically ensures you're getting a varied diet. Also, many experts claim that our bodily systems are set up for and respond well to seasonal foods.

- If you find yourself making the same dishes over and over again, peruse the Internet for new raw vegan recipes, get an app, attend a class or purchase a book. I find these activities inspiring and they often give me just the little nudge I need to get out of a rut. However, if you're like me and tend to *enjoy* eating one dish for weeks on end, you can do that! How? To ensure you are continually getting a good variety of nutrients even if you're making the same dish repeatedly, simply rotate your ingredients. Say you're stuck on lettuce tacos. If you continually change up the kind of lettuce, toppings, or nut/seed pâté, you're sure to be treating yourself to a wide variety of nutritious foods.

- Stopping by a local farmers' market may result in the discovery of a new fruit, veggie, nut or seed you haven't yet tried. Figuring out how to incorporate different foods into your meal plan can infuse new life into an old routine.

- Include fermented foods! These are amazing for promoting healthy gut flora and I love the taste! I include simple kombucha and sauerkraut recipes for you in the recipe section.

- Create new sauces, dips or dressings and use them with old staples, such as the faithful salad, spiralized cucumber "spaghetti," or crackers (we'll discuss the raw version of crackers and bread later).

- Watch your sugar intake, including what you'll get from dried fruit and so on, but you *can* eat dessert for breakfast, lunch, snacks or dinner! There are no hard and fast rules here, and as everything you're going to be consuming is actually healthy food, go to town! My two warnings here are:

- Eating heavily (nuts and seeds or breads, etc.) too late in the evening can result in all-night digestion instead of restful and restorative sleep. A smoothie or light dinner consumed not *too* late in the evening can have you waking up rested and refreshed instead of sluggish.

- Over-consuming sugar (a common raw vegan mistake) can result in weight gain, skin issues and less-than-optimal health.

- Try some new herbs or spices. These offer a variety of health benefits and can really, um, spice up your diet!

- Invite a friend or two over and try out a new dish. Creating delicious food can be a really enjoyable way to spend an evening and leave you with leftovers to eat later.

Alright, now on to the actual food.

Below I've listed some typical, easy, go-to meals. These are the heavy hitters I tend to go back to over and over again. I've also included simple options for mixing things up and some scaled-down versions for the "I've got no food at home!" days.

Note: all nuts and seeds are soaked and/or sprouted (see the nut and seed section below for easy how-to instructions).

Juices and Smoothies

Smoothies and juices are often mistaken for one another, but are actually completely different items. A juicer extracts the juice from the fruit or vegetable, separating the pulp/fiber from the liquid. A smoothie, however, is created in a blender using the entire food; thus the pulp/fiber is retained and blended together with the juice. There are benefits to both beverages, and I highly recommend including both in your healthy diet.

A note about fiber: As you first start to eat more raw food, I suggest including lots of fiber. Fortunately, this is super easy to do and almost unavoidable when eating whole, raw foods. Fiber will assist in the detoxification process; like a brush, fiber actually cleans toxins out of the body. For this reason, if you've got to choose one over the other—smoothie or juice—I'd go with the smoothie at first. As a raw foodist, you don't really have to think about how to get fiber or take a supplement; fiber is just naturally included in your regular diet. (I was once astonished to see a popular T.V. doctor recommend a fiber supplement and completely neglect to mention the easy step of increasing your intake of fiber-rich foods! I guess it was all about the product sales . . .) At first, people who aren't used to much fiber, may experience digestive difficulty, including bloating and gas. If this is the case, don't hesitate to lean more heavily on juices rather than smoothies at first, and then slowly introduce more fiber as you go along.

Juices and smoothies share many benefits because they both:

- Easily incorporate fresh fruits and veggies into the diet.

- Retain most of the vitamins, minerals, antioxidants and phytonutrients found in whole versions of foods. These natural substances protect against cardiovascular disease, cancer and inflammatory diseases, to name a few.

- Digest easily.

- Reduce cravings for other foods.

I think of a smoothie as more of a full meal, and in fact will often whip one up for a super-easy dinner, while I enjoy juices as nutrient-dense beverages.

Drinking juices and smoothies alone, rather than combining them with other foods, allows the body to more readily absorb the nutrients, thereby reaping the full benefits of these drinks.

With both juices and smoothies, I use a basic recipe that I then vary with the seasons and with available produce. As a rule, I do not use fruit in my juices. Eating whole fruit separately allows the fiber in the fruit to slow the absorption of the naturally occurring sugars. I do use a *small* amount of fruit in my smoothies however, as the fiber is retained. Primarily I juice and blend green vegetables, as you'll note below.

Tip: As previously mentioned, I keep all of my juicing and smoothie ingredients in a basket (or separate drawer) in my fridge. Making one or the other is a breeze—I just pull out the correct ingredient container and get going!

Second tip: I commissioned a seamstress to sew various sized bags out of flour sack dishtowels. I store all of my refrigerated veggies in these bags, which I keep damp either by running them under cool water prior to filling them and/or by periodically spraying them with water from a small spray bottle kept in the fridge door. These bags are simple to maintain (I toss them in the washer and dryer frequently), and keep plastic away from your foods. They also keep the veggies crisp and nice for much longer, and you may even notice that with these bags your fridge will take on a quiet calmness that plastic does not seem to afford. They can also be used as produce bags at the store, helping to eliminate plastics from the environment.

Juices

Equipment: Juicer

Base: My juice base almost always includes the following:

1–2 cucumbers
3–4 carrots (optional for sweetness)
1 bunch of kale (depending on size) or other dark leafy greens (chard, spinach, collard greens, etc.)
3 stalks of celery

Everything else is up for grabs.

Note: As mentioned, I will typically juice a full juice container-sized batch (4 cups or so) and split this into two juices, one of which gets refrigerated for the next day.

Additional content: I juice whatever arrives that week in my CSA box and add health-boosting goodies like watercress, carrot or beet greens, celery root, ginger, turmeric, beet, burdock, cayenne, mustard greens, tomatoes, cabbage, broccoli, cauliflower, radish and, rarely, apple. I love the option of juicing items I don't like to eat raw. Broccoli, for example, though I used to love it steamed, does not usually appeal to me raw. So I juice it! I will juice just about anything, especially if it's green!

Sweetener: While I'm not a sweets person by any stretch, I used to find it difficult to stomach a pure green juice without any sweetness at all. I would sometimes juice an apple or a quarter of a beet if that ended up in my kitchen, but any more than that and I had the dreaded sugar high. Ugh. And while some will advise against juicing *any* root item at all for this very reason, I found that I did fine with a few carrots, and I like the taste. More recently, however, I've found I prefer to simply juice the greens and leave out the sweetener completely.

Emergency juice: When I'm out of my juice-base items I'll just juice up whatever I've got. Unless it's all carrots, apples, beets or other too-sweet items, any juice is better than no juice in my book!

Health note: Juices are powerhouses of nutrition and can have many benefits. A full discussion is beyond the scope of this book, but a reference like Balch's *Prescription for Natural Healing* is great for exploring the many health benefits of veggies, fruits and more.

Smoothies

Equipment: High-powered blender

How: Add all ingredients and blend to desired consistency

Base: The base for my smoothie is so important to me that if I don't have the base items, I will probably skip my smoothie until I can get to the store. This is because I'm a texture tyrant! Texture is more important to me than taste, although there's no reason not to have both. I like my smoothies on the thin side, fully emulsified. Chunks and strings are gag-inducing for me, and I avoid them with a passion.

My smoothie base includes: one banana, a tablespoon or so of coconut oil and a couple handfuls of greens. There are arguments against using bananas, but I draw the line there as I haven't found a texture substitute I enjoy. Others use avocado or coconut meat as a base. These are okay, albeit more expensive than banana (and in the case of coconut meat, a big step-up in effort—I have not found pre-packaged coconut meat palatable), but I prefer the texture of bananas to anything else.

Note: As previously mentioned, I will typically make a full blender container of smoothie and split this into two batches, one of which gets refrigerated for evening or for the next day. I use Blender Bottle containers for both my juices and smoothies. They seal tightly, are BPA-free and make it easy to re-shake at will.

Content: The content of my smoothies varies greatly from week to week. For the greens, I prefer spinach, but I'll use almost any green available, including kale, bok choy, arugula, dandelion or mustard greens (a little goes a long way here!), lettuce and collard greens. I also typically add a scoop of dried chlorella, wheatgrass or other supergreen/superfood powder. (See Chapter Twelve: Basic Nutrition and Supplementation.) You can also include an orange or grapefruit in your smoothies (be careful; grapefruit can interfere with some medications—check before consuming). As always, switching up ingredients here is oh-so-important nutritionally.

A little lemon, lime or grapefruit peel can be eaten raw and included in smoothies, although typically these are somewhat bitter. The fruit pith (white part between the fruit and peel) is quite nutritionally dense and should definitely be included if possible. Make sure to use only organic fruits—pesticides can be concentrated in the peel.

You can certainly add berries (fresh or frozen work) or other fruits as well. For extra calories, protein and healthy fats, you can add tasty nut butters or tahini.

I then add water until the smoothie is the consistency I prefer. You can also use coconut water or almond milk, but they are much pricier (and add more calories, which may or may not be a plus for you) than filtered water.

Sweetener: Banana and maybe a small orange. That's it for me. If I'm out of banana and using avocado or coconut as my base, I might throw in a pitted date or two for sweetener. If you're used to a sweeter drink than this, by all means add another banana, stevia, additional fruits or a few more dates. I do recommend cutting down on sugar as you get used to the raw diet, however, as sugar can cause issues with blood sugar levels and impact fat storage. If you want to go non-vegan and use raw honey to sweeten your smoothie, that's another option (local honey may have positive effects on those suffering from allergies as well). I recommend avoiding most other packaged sweeteners, such as agave nectar, due to their processed nature and tendency to spike blood sugar levels.

Emergency smoothie: If I'm completely out of greens (egads!), I will use a powdered greens or super greens product mixed with water. If all I have is a banana, water and super greens, I'll call that a go.

Health note: As mentioned above with juices, you can explore boosting the health benefits of your smoothies by researching different ingredients in a reference book like Balch's *Prescription for Natural Healing*.

Nuts and Seeds

The Seedling in the Sink: Soaking and Sprouting Basics

As you start diving into eating raw food, the subject of soaking and sprouting will eventually come up. I avoided soaking or sprouting for about a year after I started eating raw food, thinking this was a complex, confusing activity that I'd figure out later. I continued purchasing pre-sprouted nuts and seeds, which are often sold at ten times the price of their unsoaked, unsprouted counterparts.

Eventually, I was ready to explore soaking and sprouting. When I did, I couldn't believe how easy it was! It's *so* easy, in fact, that if a seed gets stuck in the drain of my sink, it just grows on its own; of course, these little guys are *designed* to sprout! Through trial and error, I developed what seems to me to be the simplest method, which is what I'll relay to you in a moment. But first, let's discuss why we want to soak and/or sprout in the first place.

Soaking

Nuts and seeds are beautifully designed. They've developed natural defenses to ensure their survival. One of these defenses comes in the form of enzyme inhibitors. Enzyme inhibitors are substances within nuts and seeds that ensure the survival of the seed or nut until conditions are right for growth. When a bird swallows a seed, the seed is safely passed intact through the bird's digestive system and will not sprout until conditions are right—because of enzyme inhibitors. Optimal conditions for sprouting include water, warmth, sunlight and—in the best of all possible worlds—springtime. When we soak nuts and seeds, we're providing conditions for them to sprout.

The compounds that inhibit nut and seed digestion in birds operate the same way in humans. When we eat nuts and seeds that have not been soaked, they still contain these enzyme inhibitors and are therefore difficult to digest. Not surprisingly, some people experience significant digestive issues when eating unsoaked nuts and seeds. When we soak and/or sprout nuts and seeds, the inhibitors are released and rinsed away and we can then easily digest these mini nutritional powerhouses.

Raw nuts and seeds also contain phytic acid, which serves as a protectant and antioxidant for plants. Like enzyme inhibitors, phytic acid is useful in safeguarding seeds until germination. When consumed by humans, phytic acid binds to minerals in the gastrointestinal tract, which can cause irritation and impact absorption of those minerals.

Soaking also encourages the production of beneficial enzymes and renders nutrients more readily available for absorption. Additionally, many nutrients are activated and increased (e.g., vitamins A, B and C) by the process of soaking. Soaked and dehydrated nuts and seeds have a nice, crispy texture and simply taste worlds better than the unsoaked versions. I promise you, if you get used to eating soaked nuts and seeds you will never want to go back to eating the unsoaked versions!

You can soak all of the nuts and seeds you purchase before consuming them except for flax (which will simply turn into goo) and chia (unless you want to sprout them). Pumpkin seeds, sunflower seeds, Brazil nuts, pecans and walnuts are some of my favorites. I do not recommend using peanuts in general as there are some significant issues there with toxins, inflammation and allergy. Many people (including myself) are also allergic to cashews, as they are related to poison ivy.[57]

Sprouting

You can soak and sprout almost any raw seed, as well as truly raw almonds and buckwheat (which is actually a tiny fruit). But Brazil nuts, cashews, hazelnuts, macadamia nuts, pecans, walnuts, pistachios and other nuts will not sprout.

When we sprout these little guys, the benefits of soaking still apply but we also reap some additional rewards. With sprouting, protein and fat content are altered, resulting in higher protein and lower fat composition. In general, sprouting also unlocks the nutrients in the nut or seed and anti-nutrients (compounds that block mineral absorption) are disabled.

Sprouts can become vulnerable to contamination, leading to bacterial overgrowth that may result in food-borne illnesses, so just keep your little sprouts clean and fresh, and eat them ASAP out of the fridge, or dehydrate at a low temperature; this allows them to retain most of their nutritional value.

As mentioned, soaking and sprouting your own nuts and seeds as opposed to purchasing them pre-sprouted will save you a *lot* of cash. In addition, packaged nuts and seeds may also contain salt, of which I'm not a huge fan. If *you* are, sea salt can be a great option to add yourself.

A quick note on legumes and grains: many people eating a raw food diet soak and sprout both legumes and grains. I tend to find these difficult to digest and unpleasant to eat. The exception is when I visit one of my favorite restaurants, Au Lac, in Fountain Valley and downtown Los Angeles, California. Chef Ito uses sprouted rice routinely in their dishes, which are delectable and give me no digestive issues whatsoever. They do, however, feel a bit heavy to me, and so I limit my grain consumption to those cherished trips to Au Lac.

I have soaked and fermented wild rice myself, and it is delicious. However, even wild rice goes through a heat process (parching) before it gets to the store and is very difficult to find truly raw. Because I'm extremely sensitive to the difference in the energetic feeling of raw versus cooked food once I've eaten it, I do not like the heavy feeling of wild rice and in general prefer not to eat rice at all.

Now let's look at the how-to of soaking and sprouting.

How to *Soak* Nuts and Seeds

Soaking is the simplest thing in the world:

1. Purchase organic, raw nuts/seeds. Roasted and/or pasteurized nuts and seeds are dead and will not grow.

2. Place nuts/seeds into a large, lead-free container (I like to use glass mixing bowls, salad bowls or fruit bowls). Make sure there is enough room for them to absorb water and expand. You can also pour your nuts/seeds into a nut mylk bag prior to placing them in the container of water. This simplifies the job of rinsing them when they're done soaking as you can simply hold the bag under the stream of water.

3. Cover completely with filtered water.

4. Add sea salt: Though I didn't add this step for years, some sources advise adding approximately 1 tablespoon of sea salt to every four cups of nuts. The salt assists in deactivating enzyme inhibitors.

5. Cover dish and let sit overnight. I often use a plate or small cutting board as a lid.

   Soaking Time: There is an incredible variety of different nuts and seeds (and grains and legumes, if you want to go there as well). Instead of listing the soaking and sprouting times for each, which of course you can look up online if you want to, here are a couple of general rules: Soak all nuts and seeds for 8–12 hours. Though some need less, if you just remember 8–12 hours, this will cover your soaking times, with the exception of almonds, which will need to be soaked for 24–48 hours. Rice and legumes need a soak time of about 12 hours.

6. Rinse well.

7. Optional: Dehydrate. If you're not going to sprout (as noted, most nuts do not sprout), my favorite thing to do is to spread the soaked nuts/seeds out on a dehydrator tray and dehydrate below 118 degrees until fully dry. This can take a day to two, depending on how thickly you spread the nuts and seeds, and on what you're dehydrating, but is well worth the time.

8. Unless I'm preparing a recipe right away, I then pour the nuts/seeds into jars and pop them into the fridge or freezer. Most thoroughly dehydrated nuts last six months to a year in the fridge and one to two years frozen. Wet nuts and seeds in the fridge will start to mold after only a few days. If I'm going to consume the nuts/seeds fairly quickly (within three months), I often just pop them onto a shelf in a cupboard or in my pantry, as some nuts or seeds may become a bit less crispy in the fridge. If you're using a dehydrator, you can stock up on a variety of nuts and seeds to use in recipes for weeks ahead.

How to Sprout Seeds and Nuts

Sprouting takes a bit more effort than merely soaking, but not much. It also takes longer: sprouting can take up to five days, but you will be able to see tiny sprouts any time before that with most seeds. After you've soaked your nuts/seeds, the idea is to provide the little guys with the proper conditions for growth. You can use buckwheat or almost any seed, although sunflower seeds, chia and quinoa sprout very quickly and are some of my favorites. There are several ways to sprout. Some people use glass jars, some plant the seeds in soil, and some use specifically designed sprouting devices. I've found that the easiest way to sprout is to use nut mylk bags, which can be purchased online for around eight bucks. Whole Foods (and I'm sure others) also sells inexpensive mesh produce bags that work nicely. If using buckwheat, for instance, your final sprouts will be about double the size of your initial buckwheat, so leave room in the nut mylk bag!

Here's how to do it:

1. After nuts/seeds have been soaked and rinsed, place them in the nut mylk bag, or simply start out with them in the bag. Either procedure is fine, but I particularly like to place very small seeds or buckwheat in the nut mylk bag prior to soaking and soak them in the bag. Rinsing is then quite simple and is done by running water over the seeds/nuts while they are inside the nut mylk bag. Do not remove from bag after soaking.

2. Water the bag. Make sure to slosh water over all of the nuts and seeds while they're in the bag. Using filtered water is ideal.

3. Hang the nut mylk bag. I have a hook on the cabinet next to my sink and I place a bowl underneath the bag so it doesn't drain all over the counter. Squish the bag around as you water it a few times a day so that all of the nuts/seeds stay wet and clean.

4. Watch for sprouts to appear (typically within one to three days, but this may take up to five days for some seeds).

5. Grow sprouts to desired length (one quarter to half an inch is fine), continuing to rinse/water the plants a few times a day.

6. Eat, place in fridge or freezer, or arrange sprouts in dehydrator and dry. Dehydrating *can* minimally affect nutrients, although low-heat dehydration (under 118 degrees) results in very little nutrient loss and exponentially increases the amount of time you can store your sprouts.

Nut and Seed Pâtés

Nut and seed pâtés are astonishingly easy to prepare and are almost always part of my weekly raw arsenal. I lean more on the seed than the nut side, as seeds tend to be higher in protein and lower in fat, although I also use nuts and don't tend to worry about the fat content. My body tells me what it prefers and I do very well eating nuts. We need healthy fats! I particularly love walnuts and pecans. Diets that include nuts have been noted to be longevity-friendly.

Pâtés are extremely versatile. You can stuff a red pepper (or any pepper) with pâté and slice it in half, fill small mushroom caps, create lettuce-leaf tacos or fill an avocado half or portobello mushroom. The sky's the limit!

Equipment: Food processor

How: Simply place ingredients in a food processor and grind to desired consistency. I like my pâtés slightly chunky so that I can still identify most of the ingredients, rather than ground to a paste-like consistency. To each his own.

Base: Any nut or seed. Sunflower seeds are one of my favorites; they're cheap, packed with protein and versatile. I also like to use pumpkin seeds, almonds, pecans, Brazil nuts, etc. While cashews are very versatile and nothing compares to their creaminess (particularly for sauces and desserts), as mentioned, they are a member of the poison ivy family. I'm often visited by nifty little rashes if I consume cashews, so pay attention for that in case you happen to be allergic yourself.

Content: I will often add spices, seaweed, tomatoes, nutritional yeast, green onions, parsley, bell pepper, cilantro, coconut aminos (see Supplements section) and/or miso paste to my pâtés. You can pretty much add whatever appeals to you. I almost always add a couple of teaspoons of olive oil for texture. My all-time favorite pâté is "taco meat" made with walnuts, coconut aminos, olive oil, and a little red pepper flake. Adding nutritional yeast will result in a delicious cheesy flavor.

Seasoning: Seasoning is key! If you're using aminos or miso paste, these are very tasty in themselves, but I often also add one or more of the following to my pâtés: red pepper flakes, turmeric, basil, sea salt, black pepper, curry, poultry seasoning (one of my favorites), etc. Mix it up with different spices, but buy organic!

Emergency pâté: Emergency pâté is so easy! Take any nut or seed, toss in a couple tablespoons of oil and whatever seasoning you've got on hand, blend it in the food processor to desired consistency, and you're done and done!

Health note: The world of spices is a cornucopia of healing wealth. Each spice imparts individual health benefits and its own nutritional profile. I encourage you to research specific spices to address issues you might be facing, and to then add them liberally to your next pâté.

Nut and Seed Mylks

Nut and seed mylks are yet another raw food item that seemed overwhelming to me at first. Actually, they could not be easier. I made nutritious nut mylk for the baby on a daily basis in addition to nursing.

Equipment: High speed blender, nut mylk bag, container for mylk, container for pulp.

Remember to always use your nut mylk bags with the seams facing outside. This makes them much easier to clear.

How:

1. Place any nuts or seeds in a high-speed blender and add about the same amount of filtered water. You can vary the richness of the mylk by adjusting the amount of water used. Less water equals a richer mylk.

2. Blend until you no longer hear the clicking of the nut fragments against the blender container. But stop as soon as the clicking does! Do not blend too long or you'll have a heck of a time squeezing the mylk out of the fine-sand pulp. You'll get a feel for this as you go along.

3. Position your nut mylk bag over the container that the mylk will go into. I often use a glass measuring pitcher; you want something the mouth of the nut mylk bag will completely cover if possible.

4. Pour your nut mylk and pulp through the nut mylk bag.

5. Squeeze the mylk from the pulp in the bag.

6. Empty the pulp into a container and use immediately (it's a great cookie base!) or refrigerate/freeze for future use.

7. Some like to add a bit of sweetener to their mylk; my favorite is a date or two. This can be done by adding the separated mylk and the sweetener/date back into the blender and emulsifying.

There's no end to the various mylk concoctions you can create by adding vanilla, nutmeg or other spices, for example. Chai flavor, chocolate milk or egg-nog can be whipped up in a jiffy. Voilà! An easy, nutritious, delicious beverage!

Cereals

Cereal can serve as a yummy breakfast, lunch, snack or dinner, and is easy to pack for travel. I love raw cereal! The cereals I make tend to be filling and calorie dense, but if you don't mind that, have at it.

Equipment: Food processor

How: Dump in ingredients and blend slightly, but leave raisins for last and stir in so that they remain whole.

Base: The base of my cereals is usually buckwheat. I love buckwheat! And as I mentioned earlier, contrary to its name, buckwheat is actually a tiny fruit. SO cute! My body does well with buckwheat and I find it indispensable as a healthy "bulkifier" or filler and for making bread and often crackers. It also sprouts quickly, is nutritionally dense and really inexpensive.

Content: Whatever nuts or seeds you have on hand. Soaked and sprouted quinoa (use your nut mylk bag for sprouting quinoa) can be good too. I usually use about half mixed nuts/seeds and half buckwheat. I sometimes also use spices, dried coconut or cacao nibs/powder to make it a bit zippier. Chia seeds and ground flax seeds are great, although these will thicken the cereal when liquid is added. Ground flax will also go rancid quickly. I tend to go light on the flax for this reason—well, that and its tell-tale slimy texture. I usually save the flax for my protein bars. I will sometimes blend or mix in bits of dehydrated apple or other fruit and almost always stir in whole raisins after blending the main ingredients.

You can use nut or seed mylks over the cereal, or simply use filtered water like I do. It may sound gross, but I actually like it.

I love to cut up a piece of fresh fruit to beautify and add a burst of flavor and nutrients to my cereal (pear, apple, banana and peach are terrific), or I'll add a handful of berries (blueberries are great) before digging in.

Seasoning: My favorites are nutmeg and cinnamon, but if you have another favorite seasoning, go for it.

Emergency cereal: Even without buckwheat, grinding up whatever nuts and/or seeds you have and adding a spice or two can make a solid cereal. Pour a little water over it and you're good to go.

The easiest cereal of all is a bowl of chia seeds soaked in water with a sliced banana over it. I love adding cinnamon and nutmeg to this as well. This is a great travel option as bananas and chia are easy to carry, and both can usually be purchased at major grocery chains these days. I am currently obsessed with a cereal mix that resembles a Cream of Wheat texture and is made of chia seeds, hemp seeds, protein powder, tahini, vanilla, raisins and cut up fruit mixed well with warm water. I mix the dry ingredients and keep them in a bag in the fridge. Easy. Yum.

Protein Bars

Protein bars are super simple to whip up and are great travel companions. I try to always have a batch of these on hand to take with me wherever I go during a typical week, and they're often a meal staple on my longer trips. They're usually one of my go-to between-meal snacks at home or on the road.

Equipment: Food processor, dehydrator with Teflex sheets

How: Roughly blend ingredients in processor and spread onto a Teflex sheet in the dehydrator; an angled spatula works well for this task. Score into bar shape (use plastic or wood—metal will scratch the Teflex). Dehydrate overnight or all day till desired texture. I always break pieces off to see how moist the inside is and dehydrate until the bar is fairly dry all the way through.

Base: My protein bar base is bananas (one or two) with buckwheat (about two cups) and I also use a binder in addition to banana so the bars don't become crumbly piles of dry stuff. Flax or chia seeds work well as binders, but a word of caution: don't use more than about a third of a cup of flax or you'll get slime-bars. Trust me. A tablespoon or so of psyllium husk also works quite well as a binder.

Content: Go hog wild with protein bars! Refer to the contents of cereal above, as this is typically what I'll use in a batch of protein bars. I like to add blueberries to the tops of the bars after I've scored them so the berries look cute and stay whole on top of the bars, but if you're gentle, you can fold the blueberries in right before you pour onto the Teflex sheet. Fresh out of the dehydrator, protein bars are the bomb.

Seasoning: Same as cereal: cinnamon, nutmeg, and whatever else floats your boat.

Emergency bars: Two bananas, a bunch of buckwheat, some nuts or seeds and seasoning will suffice. Nuts and bolts for sure, but it will still hold you over till your next meal.

Simple Wraps

I use wraps to make "tacos" at least once or twice almost every week (sometimes a lot more often than that). Whole, de-veined chard, butter lettuce, iceberg lettuce and collard greens also make great "tortillas" as well. These wraps quickly became staples for me as they are super-quick entree items and you can pack them up to go or enjoy them at home.

Equipment: None

How: I use a lettuce leaf as a wrap quite often, or half of a chard leaf. It's pretty self-explanatory: I simply fill the clean leaf with a pâté, add toppings (tomato, avocado, nutritional yeast, green onions, etc.), wrap it up and I'm on my way, no fuss, no muss! Okay there *might* be some muss: pack a napkin too!

If you want to get fancy, you can easily prepare tortillas by food processing up a bunch of spinach or other greens, a couple of tablespoons of psyllium husk, a dash of oil, and a bit of lemon juice until well-mixed. Add any spices you like as well. I will typically add a bit of sea salt and perhaps some cayenne if I'm feeling spicy. Pour and spread tortilla-shaped rounds onto Teflex sheets (making them as thin as possible without holes) and dehydrate until you can peel the round off the sheets without tearing them (a few hours—make sure they're still flexible, but if dehydrated too long, I use them as a tostada crisp). These are divine, and so handy.

Alternatively, you can buy premade wraps: Paleo Wraps (made of coconut) and WrawP's (more like a thin bread) are my very favorites.

Cinnamon Raisin Bread

Sometimes I find that I'm just craving a cozy little loaf of bread, so I make one! Although it's somewhat dense and not altogether like cooked bread, I've become very fond of these little loaves.

Equipment: Food processor, dehydrator

How: Dump ingredients into the food processor and blend slightly. Leave raisins for last and stir in so that they remain whole. After I've blended everything and stirred in the raisins, I form it into loaves and place on the mesh dehydrator tray for several hours. Dividing into smaller loaves decreases dehydrating time. Sometimes I'll spread a little coconut oil on a piece before tucking in, and then eat it warm directly out of the dehydrator.

Base: 1–2 bananas, 3 dates (or more if you like it sweeter), 1 cup of nuts or seeds (I like sunflower), 1 tbsp psyllium husk, enough water to give it a bread-like texture, and 2–3 cups buckwheat.

Content: I'll sometimes add carrots or anything else that strikes my fancy. Adding some olive oil gives the edges a crispy texture, which I really like.

Spices: Cinnamon and/or nutmeg. A splash of vanilla can also be a great addition.

TIP: For the best raw bread I've ever had, check out Laurel Anderson's *Wild Plate,* a beautiful book with gorgeous photos and super-amazing recipes.

Desserts

Berry Delight: In the summer, one of my most treasured treats is berries covered in nut or seed mylk with a dollop of an easy, slightly sweetened nut cream. Delish!

Raw ice cream: Banana ice cream is a raw standard; simply peel and freeze bananas and then blend in the food processor to desired consistency—so good! Can be eaten plain or add cacao, tahini, fruit, vanilla, or anything else that appeals to you. Warning: this doesn't keep well in the fridge or freezer, so just make as many servings as you'll eat right away. I will usually eat one banana's worth at a sitting.

Cookies: I often spin up some almond pulp with a couple of dates and some cacao nibs in the food processor, roll it into balls and enjoy a very simple rendition of cookies. You can play with ingredients and flavors, or also try dehydrating for a slightly different experience.

Kombucha

Kombucha is an excellent and tasty way to include fermented foods (and thus beneficial bacteria) in your diet. I drink a cup nearly every morning and substitute a fancy wine glass full of kombucha for those times when I used to enjoy a glass of wine many moons ago.

I tend to prefer plain rather than flavored kombucha, but you can get as fancy and creative with flavors as you'd like. I've set up a little "fermentation station" in my kitchen, which consists of a small four-shelf metal rack that holds all of my kombucha and sauerkraut supplies as well as the brewing delicacies themselves. Having everything in one place makes the process easy and fairly quick as well, and I almost always have batches of both brewing.

One of the beauties of fermented food (as with soaking, sprouting and dehydrating), is that while they take a little planning ahead, the actual work is done while you sleep, run errands or otherwise go about your life. Kombucha is only initially complicated by the need to procure a "scoby" (Symbiotic Culture of Bacteria and Yeast) prior to starting your first batch. Your scoby is a gelatinous round of coagulated goo and will quickly procreate. Soon you can provide friends and family with starter kits—one of my favorite gifts to give! A scoby can be ordered online or by purchasing a store-bought kombucha (you must use a raw, unflavored one) and nurturing and growing one yourself; I explain how to do this in the "How" section below.

Equipment: Gallon glass jars (I use old pickle jars and have also ordered jars online from Uline—you will need at least two, and if also making sauerkraut, I recommend obtaining at least 4; they are also great for dehydrated nut/seed storage), 1-cup measuring cup, wooden or plastic stirring spoon, funnel if adding flavors and/or transferring to smaller bottles. Make sure everything you use (including your hands) is extremely clean, but not soapy, which your scoby will hate. I don't use soap on my kombucha jars—I sterilize them with boiling water before their first use and then rinse them with hot water between uses.

Ingredients: Scoby, raw sugar, black tea (you can also substitute up to 50% green tea, but make sure you use at least 50 percent black tea). I purchase boxes of tea from Whole Foods rather cheaply.

How:

1. Brew sun tea. Fill the gallon jar with filtered water to the neck where it starts to curve inward. Add 8 teabags to water (you'll need to leave enough room for your scoby and for 2 cups of previously brewed kombucha after the tea is made). Don't

worry about caffeine or too much sugar (both of which I avoid like the plague); the scoby feeds on both. Let sit for a couple of days in or near a window.

2. Remove tea bags (squeeze out into tea) and add a cup of raw sugar. I like to use raw coconut sugar. Mix until as dissolved as possible.

3. Gently, by scooping it up with your hand and lightly "taco-folding," place your scoby on top of the tea. Your scoby will most likely float on top, although sometimes it may choose to lounge sideways or sit at the bottom, which is fine too.

   Note: If growing your own scoby from store-bought kombucha, simply put the scoby and kombucha into the jar after Step 2 and leave it alone for a month (see Step 6). Then start again at Step 1 to create your first batch of Kombucha.

4. Add two cups of previously made kombucha, either from prior batches or from a store-bought bottle (again, use only raw and unflavored).

5. Place a coffee filter secured by a rubber band over the top. This keeps bugs and unwanted particles of stuff from getting in there.

6. Place in a dark, protected, warm-as-possible area. In winter, after wrapping the jars in old towels, I snuggle my kombucha bottles in soft-sided coolers before placing them on their shelves and covering the entire shelving unit with a blanket.

7. Taste after a few days. Your kombucha will be a beautiful golden brown (the more green tea used, the lighter the color will be) and taste a bit fizzy. Leave until the sweetness is as you like it. I prefer mine almost vinegar-like, so I leave it for a while. Kombucha will brew more quickly in warmer temperatures, so check it more frequently if warm. (If you

leave it too long, simply refrigerate and use as vinegar—a little in your morning water is fantastic).

8. When kombucha is brewed to desired taste, remove your scoby and two cups of kombucha and place them in another jar to rest (my friend calls this her "scoby hotel"). Rubber band another coffee filter over the top. This will be ready to start your next kombucha batch.

9. Place kombucha in the fridge to halt the fermentation process and cover it with a lid. Enjoy!

Note: Scobys are living organisms and are said to respond well to positive treatment. I talk sweetly to my scobys and they always provide me with wonderful kombucha. Happy scoby equals happy drinks! A scoby is happy and healthy when it's whitish-tan. If you see mold (black or green spots), it's time to start over. Other irregularities are generally fine. Use your best judgement and/or take a look at photos online.

Flavorings: After your kombucha is brewed to your liking, you can choose to allow for a second ferment and add flavors, such as fresh mint, lime, blackberries, ginger or peach (don't ginger and peach sound terrific together?). Simply bottle your fresh kombucha in small glass drinking bottles (you will probably need a funnel for this), such as Perrier bottles. Add the preferred flavorings and let them sit for a few days out of direct sunlight at room temperature. No scoby required for this stage. Strain and enjoy! Alternately, you can toss your flavorings directly into your final kombucha in the fridge. The flavorings don't tend to infuse as strongly with this method, but it's quick and easy.

Sauerkraut

Sauerkraut is another one of my favorite probiotic foods. I love adding it to tacos and wraps. I also enjoy it as a side dish or just eat a few forkfuls on its own. I make a very basic sauerkraut that's super easy to prepare. It's also really beautiful, and if you use both green and purple cabbage it looks a lot like rose petals when served.

Equipment: Gallon glass jars (you can use smaller jars if you'd like of course; I like to get it all done in one fell swoop), knife, cutting board (or alternatively, food processor with or without a shredding blade can be used)

Base: Cabbage (I layer purple and green), sea salt

How:

1. Sterilize jar with boiling water.

2. Wash and peel off the outer leaves of the cabbage. Set aside.

3. Shred your cabbage. I use about 4 heads and either cut them up with a knife or shred them with the food processor. I prefer the texture of knife-prepared cabbage, but if I'm in a hurry, I'll use the processor.

4. Place the cabbage in a bowl and sprinkle liberally with salt.

5. Knead the cabbage so that it starts to soften and release water. Place the kneaded cabbage and any liquid into the gallon jar, tamping it down with your fist as you go. The goal is to squish out any air pockets in the cabbage and to cover it in its own juice.

6. Continue adding cabbage until the jar is almost full. Keep tamping forcefully (this can be quite a workout) until the cabbage is covered in liquid and no air pockets remain.

7. Place the outer cabbage leaves over the top of your shredded cabbage.

8. Weigh the top down so that the cabbage will stay submerged. Many people use a stone or other heavy object. I've found that inverting a shot glass and then screwing the lid of the jar down on top of it does the trick quite nicely.

9. Place in a dark area (I use my fermentation station) and let your cabbage sit for a week or so.

10. When it tastes the way you like it, refrigerate and enjoy!

Flavors: As with kombucha, you can flavor your cabbage by adding additional ingredients, such as carrot, radish or jalapeño (one of my favorite additions!). Kimchi is easily made raw as well, and additional recipes for all kinds of fermented foods can be found online.

♥ ♥ ♥

I hope it's apparent after this chapter that although eating raw may involve a learning curve at first, it's very simple to prepare easy dishes and rotate ingredients so that you're getting a variety of nutritious and healthy foods. As you get further into your journey, finding and creating new dishes can become a rewarding pastime. I find that working in the kitchen, when I have time to do so, is therapeutic and something I look forward to. When I don't have much time for food preparation, raw food is the perfect partner; grazing on nuts, seeds, fruits and veggies is as simple as it gets.

I hope you enjoy learning to make the basics I've described here and then take things further on your own, customizing your personal menu for your unique tastes and lifestyle.

Chapter Seven

Where to Buy Your Food

Food Suggestions: Big Picture

There are so many food-shopping options in our modern world that things can get pretty confusing. But if you know what you're looking for (and you will), you can locate edible options in almost any market.

Some stores will require less work on your part as they've done much of your research for you and generally offer wholesome options. Whole Foods and Thrive Market (online) are two of these.

Will it cost more to eat healthy food? Maybe. It depends on what you're spending and how you're currently eating. But consider this: you're worth what healthy food costs. If you're going to cheap-out on something, my suggestion is not to make it food. The material your body uses to create itself on a daily basis is important stuff, and feeling great is certainly worth a few bucks more for groceries every month.

Quality, quality, quality.

Grocery Stores

Many mainstream grocery stores now recognize that there's a

market for organic foods and stock their shelves accordingly. Check out your local haunts and see if they can accommodate some or all of your new regimen. If that works, great! If not, or if you're just looking for a little more variety, the following stores carry healthy, high-quality organic foods and may be available in your area or online.

Erewhon Organic Grocer and Cafe

Although Erewhon is only available in the L.A. area, I have to mention it. In my opinion, Erewhon is the king of grocery stores, carrying only organic, high-quality foods and products. They state, "We strive to sell only the purest, ethically and sustainably produced foods, wellness and beauty products, and household items." I can always count on an array of fresh juices, elixirs and raw deli items: pizza, wraps and Thai kelp noodles for example, and all kinds of desserts. While somewhat pricey, there's never any question about quality at Erewhon.

Whole Foods Market

Whole Foods typically carries high-quality foods and used to be pretty close to Nirvana for many raw foodists. Since its acquisition by Amazon, however, I seem to notice fewer specialty items in stock.

Note that Whole Foods' products vary quite a bit from store to store. Some have great "raw" sections (prepackaged raw foods).

Whole Foods sells products which they deem to be "natural."[58] They also keep a focus on animal welfare, as well as carrying environmentally-friendly and ecologically-responsible products. They have made a commitment to voluntarily label all GMO-containing products. See their website for the full criteria used in stocking products.

While no company is perfect, I appreciate the mission of Whole Foods to bring healthy products to the public that we can generally feel good about purchasing. Whole Foods regularly partners with a variety of community programs and donates to food banks and shelters as well. Amazon is making efforts to offer healthy products at lower prices for Whole Foods customers.

Thrive Market

Thrive Market is a membership-based online store. They carry many of the same non-perishable products that Whole Foods does, but at discounted rates. Thrive describes their mission as:

> Thrive Market is a membership community that uses the power of direct buying to deliver the world's best healthy food and natural products to our members at wholesale prices, and to sponsor free memberships for low-income American families.

Thrive donates a free membership to a low-income family for every paid membership. How awesome is that? Thrive keeps an eye focused on sustainability, and the company currently offers recipes and a great little magazine. Their website is also full of how-to videos about food, lifestyle and other issues of interest.

I use Thrive Market about once a month and order items I'd normally purchase at Whole Foods or a local health food store/co-op (e.g., coconut oil, powdered superfoods, supplements). Thrive, and markets like it, can be a boon to those living in areas without access to a market carrying natural products.

Trader Joe's

While Trader Joe's certainly doesn't share the same mission that Whole Foods does, they offer some certified organic produce and focus on keeping products reasonably priced. Although I find TJ's great for certified organic fruits and some veggies, I often don't find the leafy greens to be all that great. They also provide little to no local produce; products are often flown in from all over the world.

TJ's also sells marked-down, name-brand products under their own label, but they do not reveal the original product names due to secrecy agreements with name-brand companies. Because of these agreements it's often difficult to determine where a TJ's food originated from; many packages simply reference where the food was packed. However, to keep their prices low, they do purchase straight from the supplier when they can.

TJ's also carries and labels some vegan foods, and they provide a list of their gluten-free and vegan products online. Somewhat confusingly, TJ's privately labels some of their own organic items. This means that these privately-labeled "organic" products are not verified or certified as such by the USDA and are therefore not covered under the legal definition of "organic."

TJ's official GMO statement is: "Trader Joe's Products are sourced from Non-GMO ingredients. When developing products containing ingredients likely to come from genetically modified sources, we have the supplier of the product perform the necessary research to provide documentation that the suspect ingredients are from non-GMO sources . . . In addition to this work done in developing a given item, we conduct random audits of items with potentially suspect ingredients, using an outside, third-party lab to perform the testing."

This is certainly a step in the right direction, even if TJ's does not appear to use an industry standard organization such as the Non-GMO Project to label its products as "non-GMO." This, they write, is because "there are no clear guidelines from the US governmental agencies covering food and beverage labeling. Instead of waiting for such guidelines to be put into effect, and based upon customer feedback, we took a more holistic approach and made the non-GMO ingredients position part of what the Trader Joe's label encompasses." [59]

So TJ's is a mixed bag for me. It has a fun atmosphere and some good deals on healthy foods. On the other hand, there's a lot of over-packaging of products and a lack of transparency (or at best an informal, "self-certified" status) regarding GMOs, some organic products and sourcing.

Food Co-ops and Health Food Stores

My favorite! These can be a bit spendy, but if you're able to hit farmers' markets or get CSA boxes (see the sections below) for the majority of your produce, a co-op is a great place to fill in the gaps and support the local economy while getting great quality foods.

A co-op can look like any other store (although various models exist). What makes a co-op different is that its customers can also become members who share in the ownership of the store. As an owner, you have a vote, and thus a say, in the store's business decisions.

A co-op often returns its surplus revenue to its members in proportion to how often they use the store. It may charge a reasonable membership fee, which is sometimes refundable if you leave the co-op.

Chain Stores such as Ralph's, Vons, Sprouts, Lassens etc.

Many supermarket chains now provide organic sections with contents that vary by geographical area. Check them out—you might be pleasantly surprised!

Beyond the Grocery Store

Community Supported Agriculture (CSA) Boxes

A revelation!

I love having local organic groceries delivered to my door— it's like the farmers' market comes to me. As a bonus, ordering a CSA box allows me to support local farms. My CSA boxes are delivered once a week, so Wednesday nights are like Christmas for me! I don't even need to be home or awake to receive the package; it's just left on my front stoop. Delivery is easily cancelled if I'm not going to be home, and many farms also offer the option of picking up the box yourself.

Farmers typically coordinate their own work with that of neighboring farms to provide a varied, year-long selection of produce. I love opening that box and discovering the most delicious, local, organic, seasonal produce imaginable. Many farms will offer other products, such as nuts and seeds or candles, hot sauce and bouquets for purchase on their site as well. There is simply no comparison between produce fresh from the farm and the stuff that arrives on trucks at the grocery store, often from across the country.

I can even customize my order to exactly what I want, although I often prefer to be surprised. I have used both Farm Fresh To You and Savraw and I love that they are continually expanding their options. An Internet search for "CSA box _____ (your town)" will let you know what's available in your area.

Local Farmers' Markets

The quality, variety and prices offered at farmers' markets are often terrific. There's also the added bonus of getting to know local growers and learning about their farming practices through friendly conversations as you pick out your produce. It's great to support local farms, which are often small, family-run businesses, in contrast to corporate contract farms.

All the same, you still want to be on the lookout for whether or not the produce you're picking out is organic. Many people assume farmers' market vendors are offering organic goods, but this isn't always the case. Unless specifically posted as such by the vendor, produce may very well be non-organic. If you're unsure, just ask!

It should be noted, too, that sellers bringing in less than $5,000 in annual sales are exempt from USDA organic regulations. Occasionally farmers may tell you they don't use synthetic pesticides but have not gone through the expensive process of organic certification for financial reasons. In such cases you'll simply have to use your best judgment.

Online Food Delivery Service (Not CSA)

If you live somewhere without immediate access to fresh organic food, you can often have it delivered to you, depending on your location and budget. Although this service usually isn't cheap, it can be well worth it. You can quickly discover the companies that offer this service in your area by doing an online search. In the L.A. area, two companies we've used quite happily are Rawvolution and Veggie Vibes. If home delivery isn't available to you, don't worry. Simply do your best and purchase the highest quality food you can. Even if you're eating a fresh, non-organic, plant-based, whole-foods diet, you'll still be in a better position, and in better health, than if you were eating non-organic, processed foods.

Variety Is Key

One final note that isn't so much about where you'll be getting your food but which is vital to keep in mind while shopping: you must, must, must vary your food items so that you get a variety of nutrients in your diet. Not to mention so you don't get bored and give up.

Beware of getting stuck in a rut and making the same smoothie over and over. Getting your groceries from a number of different sources can help. For example, this is where ordering a CSA box comes in handy: the produce is always seasonal and automatically varied. But you can easily vary your food yourself by making it a habit to explore what's in season, and by rotating old standbys. Hitting farmers' markets can be another great way to add variety.

It can be difficult to provide yourself with a lot of nutritional diversity if you're exclusively shopping at big chain grocery stores; they tend to consistently carry the same popular items. But you may be able to circumvent this a bit by rotating your shopping at different chain stores instead of hitting the same one each week.

You'll find that looking for variation in your diet turns shopping into something of an adventure, if you let it. Searching for a few new items each week can be an interesting treasure hunt. It's often even more fun with a friend.

I typically shop only once per week for juicing and smoothie items and nuts and seeds, and am in and out quickly because I make my food from the same structured plan, even though I vary the ingredients. I order my staples from Thrive Market, receive my weekly CSA box and hit farmers' markets now and then. I rarely make a list unless I'm preparing a new dish, and my grocery shopping usually only takes me about half an hour.

It's very simple. First I hit the organic produce for things that didn't come in my CSA box. Next I make a trip to the bulk nuts and seeds sections and then head over to Whole Foods to pick up harder-to-find organics or supplements I can't order from Thrive Market. Done and done.

A tip: I love, love, love, the raw food recipe app by The Rawtarian.[60] It currently costs around five dollars and is well worth it. This app allows you to locate raw recipes and then creates an easy-to-use shopping list for you. Genius!

I frequently pull up Rawmazing recipes as well.[61] This is a beautiful site with a recipe library for delectable raw food concoctions. Look for some other suggestions in the Resources List at the end of this book.

Happy shopping!

Chapter Eight

Restaurants & Dining Out

Depending on where you live and what your financial situation is, restaurant dining may be a simple, enjoyable experience or a frustrating chore.

If you're Oprah, for example, it doesn't matter where you are. You can have food delivered, visit a high-end establishment, and travel with a personal chef who has access to the healthiest, highest quality food on the planet.

If you're barely scraping by and living somewhere in middle America, your options may be more limited.

In the United States, restaurant dining is an important social activity. So many of our social gatherings revolve around food. No matter what socio-economic strata you find yourself in, dining out is likely a part of your food experience. Whether it's fast food, a corner café or the fanciest bistro in town, restaurant dining permeates our culture.

The good news is you can usually dine out in a healthier way than you may be used to, and in this section I'll provide you with some helpful tips.

Raw Restaurants

First of all, if you have access to raw restaurants, this is obviously the easiest way to go. It's all kinds of fun to be able to simply point at and order virtually anything on the menu. I also consider eating at raw restaurants an important source of inspiration for expanding my own menu at home.

Raw restaurants do tend to be a bit pricey and few and far between, even in the best of circumstances, but if you live in a progressive metropolitan city, you're likely to encounter at least one or two.

Raw restaurants, like any eating establishment, vary in quality and sophistication. Some offer very simple fare while others work absolute magic with ingredients and techniques you may have never heard of. Simple fare will tend toward minimally processed, whole ingredients, such as kale salads, lasagnas and soups; these can be utterly delicious. More complex offerings at sophisticated establishments may include astonishing sauces, elaborate desserts and cryptically prepared "meats," appetizers, pastas and cheeses. These more complex dishes are often heavier and much richer than the simpler fare, and both are welcome additions to my food experience. While I certainly appreciate a fancy, rich meal every once in a while, I tend to visit the heavier food places infrequently. A few of my favorite haunts in Los Angeles are Au Lac, Lenore's (amazing cabbage and beet salads!), Plant Food & Wine, Joi Café and SunCafe Organic. Café Gratitude has winnowed down its raw food options, but still offers a few dishes for the raw food enthusiast.

Note: While the above list doesn't necessarily apply to those of you outside of California, there might be some inspiration in checking out their menus online or, as I used to do myself, plan adventurous trips to special restaurants. For example, our family is planning to visit our favorite raw place in New York City, Quintessence, when we travel there next month.

Salad bar-type places, such as California Fresh or the relatively new franchise Grabba Green, are obviously slam-dunks. You can pile your plate high with all kinds of raw goodies and top it off with oil and lemon juice (or premade dressings as available). Beware that some ingredients may not be organic.

Some health food stores, such as Whole Foods, Erewhon or local co-ops (and even some larger traditional chain stores) also offer salad bars or other premade raw options. The more "natural" places will even include items such as chili flakes, raw nuts or seeds and liquid aminos to add to your creation. Knock yourself out!

Other Types of Restaurants

Sometimes, however, you'll find yourself in a situation in which you are not the one choosing the eatery, you're in a town with no raw restaurant, or everyone you know is tired of traipsing along with you to the one raw joint in town. It is this situation to which the following tips are directed.

But before we start, a word to the wise: loosen up your standards. Going absolutely organic is often not an option at many restaurants. Oh well. Unless you are incredibly chemically sensitive, this one meal is not going to kill you if it's not organic. My advice? Enjoy a meal with your friends and don't stress. The stress may cause you more damage than the pesticides!

Now for the tips.

- Let's start with the obvious: order a salad. Most restaurants include salad options on their menus. You'll have to read the menu carefully, however, and many times you'll want to ask for any cooked items that are often automatically included (croutons, etc.) to be removed. You can often choose a side or dinner salad with dark greens.

- Create your own salad. I have Markus Rothkranz to thank for this next resourceful tip. Scour the menu for anything raw that might be hiding back there in the kitchen. I've found that asking, "Can you please add anything raw you have on hand into my salad?" often results in a salad decorated with cooked broccoli, a limp mushroom and an onion sliver or two. Boo. It's much more productive to go through the menu yourself and request to add specific items to a salad already offered on the menu, and, voilà: you've created an amazing meal!

- You may be asked to pay an additional charge to have these items added, but I have enjoyed the most delicious salads this way!

- Ask for olive oil and lemon juice as a dressing. If a vinaigrette is offered, ask for the ingredients to make sure they haven't included any allergens.

- Order a plate of sliced raw veggies. Most restaurants will be able to supply you with this. Sometimes guacamole can also be ordered or you can mash up avocado slices as a sort of a dip.

- Lemon water is my favorite beverage when I dine out. It feels a bit fun and fancy and like an actual *drink*.

- I suggest tipping a bit extra if the wait staff has gone out of their way to provide you with an off-menu food experience.

The following tips may help at popular ethnic restaurants.

Mexican:

- Order cucumber slices instead of chips and dig into the salsa!

- I've often made a meal of a large order of guacamole and fresh veggie slices as "chips." Yum!

- Typically I skip the salad here. More often than not, unless you're at a really high-end place or a more Tex-Mex style joint, salads consist of iceberg lettuce, carrot shavings and some less-than-ripe tomatoes. Ew!

- Mexican restaurants sometimes feature a salsa bar where you can stock up on little cups of different salsas. I use these to dip cucumber, carrot, zucchini or celery slices (or whatever they have to offer me), or if I've ordered one, I douse my salad in this spicy goodness. Delicious.

- Raw cabbage or lettuce-leaf tacos! Adding some pico de gallo, guacamole and cut-up zucchini or other veggies can make for an enjoyable lunch or dinner.

Thai

- I love Thai food! Fresh veggie spring rolls are one of my favorite items. The rice paper and small amount of rice noodles often included aren't raw, but I make an exception here and eat them anyway. Same goes for the peanut sauce if I can get it gluten free. [62]

- Many times, Thai restaurants offer a garden salad that tends to be of better-quality. I've noticed that dark greens instead of iceberg will most often appear.

- Some Thai places will make you a vegan green papaya salad (meaning they leave out the fish sauce). This all depends on whether the salad is made to order or not. My sister and I discovered Bangkok Cuisine in Reno, where they made everything to order and were more than happy to whip up a number of items for me that were both raw and vegan. Delightful!

Greek:

- Greek salad is one of my favorites. Minus the feta, I can gorge on delicious cucumbers, olives, onions and other Greek delicacies for days.

- Though you're unlikely to find it except in a raw food restaurant, raw falafel is amazing. Drizzled with or dipped in a raw aioli, I can't get enough of this.

- Hummus! Normally hummus is not raw, but be sure and ask, because sometimes it is.

- Tahini is sometimes raw and a boon to add to salads, along with plain sesame seeds if those are available.

- If fresh kale salad is on the menu, ask for it without the tabbouleh, which is made of wheat and not raw.

Italian

Ooh. This is a tough one. While there are many raw Italian recipes, I find it tough to eat anything but salad at typical Italian restaurants. The good news is that the salads here can be good, including greens like arugula. Sometimes you can also order a plate of fresh fruit.

Picnic!

When it's an option, I've sometimes suggested a picnic rather than a restaurant. If everyone else is willing, this can be a fun little adventure.

If you don't already have prepared food you'd like to pack, a quick trip to most grocery stores will reveal at least a few items to fill your tummy and help make the picnic a total success.[63] Peruse the grocery store for items such as:

- Raw coconut water

- Raw kombucha

- Avocados

- Bananas

- Chia seeds (just add water and sliced fruit for a yummy and filling pudding)

- Fresh fruit and veggies to cut up. One of my favorites to pack is a melon. Add some cinnamon to sprinkle on top and enjoy this rejuvenating and self-packaged feast. Remember to bring a knife.

Even some standard grocery stores may carry some prepackaged raw items (be sure to check the label, because not all items may be raw), such as:

- Kale chips

- Hummus

- Garlic spread

- Nuts and seeds

- Protein bars

- Coconut wraps

- Flatbread

- Macaroons

- Cheesecake

- And if you're lucky, you might even find some entrees, such as raw Pad Thai, pizza, a burger, burrito or lasagna.

If you suffer from food allergies, check the ingredients for common offenders.

A picnic may ultimately cost you almost as much as eating at a restaurant, but it can also be a creative alternative and get you out into nature for a bit. Reconnect with the outdoors!

Dining as a Guest

Dining as a guest can be a bit of a tricky situation, but I've rarely found it to be a big issue.

There are three main scenarios when eating as a guest:

- The grazing party

- The formal preordered meal affair

- The intimate occasion

While each of these scenarios offers its own complications and solutions, one of the best pieces of advice I've received regarding eating as a guest comes from health and lifestyle coach Natasha St. Michael. Her sage wisdom is simply this: be gracious.

This has been a revelation to me. Wherever I go, instead of feeling guilty when I'm rejecting food others generously prepare and offer to me, I'm able to tactfully decline foods that I know will make me ill or foods I simply choose not to consume, without causing any kind of an uproar.

How to I pull this off? Easy! Whenever I'm offered food I'm going to decline, whether at a friend's house or a formal dinner, I look at it approvingly and say something like, "This looks absolutely delicious (if it does)! Thank you for preparing (or ordering) all of this yummy food! I'm eating pretty specifically right now so I'm going to pass, but wow that looks amazing!"

It's also helpful for me to keep in mind that my food is my responsibility. While I've found myself a bit frustrated once or twice at family dinners, I've just taken this as a cue to bring food that I can eat next time. Even better, I can bring ingredients and prepare food myself while the family is preparing their own dinner. This allows me to participate in the food-making rituals and also have something to eat. When possible, I like to make enough for everyone at the table to share.

Keeping these things in mind, let's look at some of the specific situations in which we may find ourselves dining as guests.

The Grazing Party

The grazing party includes events such as casual birthday parties, holidays and any other more-or-less informal celebration where food is laid out and everyone grabs a plate and fills it up. This situation is much less tricky than the formal preordered meal affair or the intimate occasion.

At the grazing party, invitees are often encouraged to supply a dish for the rest of the guests, which is a perfect excuse to bring something you yourself can eat. It's also an opportunity to get creative and try something new, or go with an old favorite you know will be a hit. Raw desserts are often crowd pleasers. An amazing salad is always welcome and can serve as your entire meal. If you're assigned a food category, such as an appetizer or main dish, you basically have unlimited raw food options to prepare.

Another plus to the grazing party is that no one is expecting you to eat one of everything, and people aren't closely observing what you're eating. No one has a stake in you eating anything in particular. Your plate is only so big, and if you fill it up with cucumber slices, cherry tomatoes and raw hummus, then so be it.

If the grazing party is a wedding or other catered event, basically the same rules apply. No need to make a big deal out of anything. Just accept whatever it is you'd like to eat and bypass the rest. I've attended weddings where I filled and refilled my plate with salad and raw veggies and responded to any comments with something to the effect of, "This salad is amazing, I can't get enough!"

The Formal Preordered Meal Affair

Of course if the event is a preordered meal affair where you're asked ahead of time to select menu options (like a wedding or graduation dinner), your choices are more limited. In such cases, you can either check the vegetarian box and do your best with the premade plate, or you can write in something like, "I'm on a salad kick and will save you the trouble of preparing anything else for me, thank you!"

On occasion in such situations I've been beyond starving and have eaten limp steamed veggies or rice, although I usually wish I hadn't. However, it isn't going to be life-threatening if you indulge in a few dead veggies.

If you do decide to eat something way outside of your preferred foods, remember to avoid anything you may be allergic to. Other than that, do your best and just move on; it's not that big of a deal and certainly not worth over-analyzing or beating yourself up over.

The Intimate Occasion

And then we have the intimate occasion. This is usually comprised of one-on-one meals, small family dinners or a few friends getting together and sharing a meal that is typically served and eaten together at a table. This may require a bit more finesse on your part.

The good news is that generally (though not always), these are going to be people who know you and have probably already accepted your "weird" food choices and may even welcome them.

If you're dining at a good friend's home, they may know how you're eating. Maybe they've even asked you what the heck they can make that you'll actually eat. In this case I almost always respond with something like, "Thanks for thinking of me! Plain fresh fruit is great, or a green salad is always amazing. Can I bring something to share with y'all as well? How about if I bring a dessert? I have this amazing chocolate mousse recipe I think you'll love!"

Plain fresh fruit and/or a plain green salad are familiar items to most people, and easy to provide. Do, however, specify "plain" and "fresh" fruit, or you may end up staring woefully down the barrel of a dish of canned peaches, a sugared-up, Cool-Whipped Jell-O mold, or a Chinese chicken salad.

Asking if you can bring something is not only courteous, but also allows you to have access to yet another dish you'll be able to eat. It's nice to eat with friends, and though sitting there with a pile of salad on your plate while everyone else bites into their steaks might feel weird at first, it's really about being with friends and not about the food. Though you may endure a bit of (hopefully) good-natured ribbing, they'll get used to your new habits soon enough.

Overcoming Awkwardness

I find that most awkward dining-as-a-guest situations typically involve you and only one or two other participants—and a food scenario wherein your host has refused your offer to bring anything. This kind and well-meaning person has painstakingly and heart-feltedly prepared something especially for you that you simply cannot eat. My mother, for example, has prepared meatloaf on more than one occasion and responded with genuine surprise when I tell her I'm so sorry but I'm just not able to partake. "But why?" she inquires. "It's *ground* meat!"

This is probably as good a time as any to note that the concept of "raw vegan food," while it may be very familiar and make solid common sense to you, is often extremely *un*familiar to others.

Some people have not even heard the term "raw vegan" and will look at you with complete confusion and ask, "What do you *eat??*" Even after describing the large variety of uncooked, plant-based foods you enjoy, you may still be met with a sideways glance and terse nod, then served anything from steamed broccoli to, well, meatloaf. It's not that people don't care about you, it's just that they are so conditioned to eating in a specific way that raw vegan is just way too far outside of their box for them to comprehend right away.

As a raw vegan myself, it's sometimes frustrating to note that in our food culture, no one blinks an eye at consuming large amounts of toxins, refined sugars and detrimental chemicals, such as are included in sodas, for example, while screaming that a mother feeding her child vegan food should warrant a visit from Child Protective Services. But it's all in what you're used to. For many folks, eating a plant-based diet may seem like the most insane thing ever. And think about it: if fast food and donuts are your staples like advertisers would like them to be, then yes, consuming plants might seem a little . . . different. To be blunt, our modern, mainstream ideas about what food is have turned *actual* natural eating on its head. The fact that it's so much weirder, in my book, to consume toxic or highly processed "food-like" items rather than whole foods, doesn't make it "normal."

I love what Alyssa Cohen says in her fantastic book, *Living on Live Foods:* "Eating fruits and vegetables is radical? But eating the inside of a cow or chewing the flesh off of the bones of chickens *isn't* radical???"

The raw vegan diet is *not* radical or extreme, but it may seem so to others just because it's not a common practice. I remember when the idea of eating raw was completely foreign to me as well!

Enjoying lunch at a raw restaurant with my non-raw but very interested and open friend Laura, she suddenly lit up with a smart epiphany that delighted us both: "I always thought you were really picky, but you're not picky at all! If it's not cooked, doesn't have poison sprayed on it and didn't come from an animal, you'll eat pretty much anything!"

She's absolutely right!

Some friends, family and acquaintances will be interested in talking with you about what you eat, and some will not. I personally couldn't care less if my hosts or the other guests want to know what I will and won't eat, but you'll find out right away who is interested and finds it a fun challenge to prepare something you'll like, and who waves you away with a "weirdo" label and plops a chicken and some biscuits on the table in front of you. I enjoy eating with these folks just as much as I do with those who go out of their way to make me a raw vegan meal. While I enjoy the *food* much more in the latter, either scenario is a welcome one for me because I'm eating with people I love. What others eat is none of my business.

Some people feel it's rude to refuse any food your host offers you, particularly in certain countries or cultures. Consequently, they'll eat whatever is put in front of them, including meat.

I'm all for mutual respect and appreciation. However, I simply won't eat anything I don't want to eat. Many foods, were I to ingest them, would make me ill very quickly, or result in other negative health outcomes I've experienced time and time again and don't choose to engage with anymore. Dairy products will send me to the bathroom for the rest of the night. Gluten causes a rash on my face or arms, not to mention stomach issues galore. Even "healthy" cooked foods like rice or steamed veggies sometimes cause me to go into such a heavy food coma that I must excuse myself for half an hour just to lie down.

Some side effects are not a huge deal, but I just don't prefer to experience them. If I eat cooked foods, for instance, I notice an annoying tendency for them to adhere to my teeth in an unpleasant film that's difficult to remove except with vigorous scraping with a toothbrush. I don't enjoy this.

The flip side of this is also true. I wouldn't want my guests to eat something *they* didn't want to eat just because I prepared it. I certainly wouldn't take it personally. Their food choices are their own and have nothing to do with me. I prefer everyone do what *they* prefer and that we just enjoy our time together.

Except with people who express a genuine, enthusiastic interest in the topic for its own sake (and/or because they love and accept you and are simply curious about your life), I recommend resisting the urge to talk with others about your food choices except to answer their questions briefly, humbly and neutrally. Allow them to form their own opinions and try not to take any of it personally. Many folks may simply want to try to disprove your reasons for your diet, often to justify their own choices. I respect their choices, and I don't enjoy or feel it's necessary to engage in heated discussions about unheated food.

Being true to myself with my food is something I don't generally compromise on. I like to feel great, and that's my prerogative. Most people just want you to be happy in their home or at a given event. I've found in just about every circumstance that with some tact and grace I can sidestep any items that aren't within my food realm, while at the same time thoroughly enjoying the time with my host and the other guests.

Eat Beforehand

Up above I mentioned that it helps me to remember that my food is *my* responsibility. So one valuable tidbit of wisdom I've learned is this:

EAT BEFORE YOU GO.

Get in the habit of keeping a bag of seeds or nuts in your purse or car, and grab a banana or prepare a smoothie before you depart. This is especially true if your host refuses your offer to bring food and you anticipate that nothing you can eat will be offered. That way, when the meal is served, you can "ooh" and "ah" over the delicious appearance of the dishes along with everyone else, but you won't have to starve or be tempted to indulge in something you'll regret later. Usually your host has spent valuable time preparing the food, and to acknowledge this is a wonderful gesture of love.

Remember also that staying true to yourself, while being appreciative of others, is also a gesture of love, and a very basic, important one at that.

Drink water with your friends and family, eat anything that's edible for you, and enjoy the company. Having eaten beforehand, you can let your hosts know how much you appreciate their work, but that you're not hungry, you're eating rather differently these days and you're sorry to inconvenience them. Make sure to help with the meal tear-down, including boxing leftovers and washing dishes if they'll let you. Participation, including conversation and togetherness, is what's important here.

Chapter Nine

How to Travel and Dine in Raw Vegan Splendor

Eating healthy food away from home can present an enormous challenge, even to the seasoned raw foodist. But traveling raw *can* be done. It can even become fairly natural. It just takes a little due diligence.

In my early days as a raw vegan, I might plan a month ahead for a three-day trip, spend an extravagant amount of money on expensive pre-packaged foods, starve, or give up and eat things that made me feel less than stellar. I experienced a lot of anxiety about how I was going to travel and eat at the same time.

Since then, years of frequent raw vegan travel trial and error have equipped me with skills that allow me to eat healthy raw vegan foods away from home with minimal effort.

On a trip to Las Vegas, while looking around at all the people eating absolute junk in the food court of a swanky hotel, I had a "light-bulb moment": what if travelers had access to healthy, affordable, raw vegan dining options—in Las Vegas hotels! Even a fresh juice stand or cart offering two or three items would be fantastic.

Then reality hit. Most people look forward to throwing caution to the wind and eating junk when they're on vacation—perhaps *especially* in Las Vegas.

But all this got me thinking. If you're used to the Standard American Diet, then eating pizza or hamburgers (i.e., junk) on vacation isn't that big of a deal; your system is already used to that kind of food. But if you've been eating raw vegan for a while, the thrill of kicking all your healthy eating habits to the curb for the length of your vacation loses its attraction. You know it will leave you feeling depleted, exhausted and sick, and that's no way to feel on vacation or on an important business trip. Much better to maintain mental clarity and physical health, right? So why not take all this raw food goodness on the road with you too?

It's Too Hard!

The biggest "why not" often comes in the form of the complaint, "It's too hard to eat healthy on the road." Addressing this requires a bit of a mental re-frame. It *can* be a challenge, but I have found through experience that I only rarely encounter any issues eating well wherever I am. I just may do it a little differently than I do at home. Here are some general outlook adjustments that will make traveling and eating raw vegan much easier.

Every Trip Is an Experiment

Think of each trip as an experiment, not something that has to go perfectly the first time around. Perhaps experiment with snacks on one trip, breakfasts on another, and so on. Life is an adventure; eating is just part of it! This travel/food business isn't a life or death thing. The absolute worst-case scenario is that you're going to eat something that makes you feel not so great for a bit. You'll recover. Not ideal, but not the end of the world either.

The less seriously we take ourselves with all of this the more fun we can have—and the more creative solutions we can dream up.

Adopt an attitude of curiosity, improvisation and play.

You're Not at Home Anymore

Let go of the idea that you're going to eat like you do at home, which is a surefire way to return from your trip frustrated and hungry. You probably won't eat identically to your regular routine, and that's okay. Variety is the spice of life, right? In many cases, you won't have access to everything you need to make fabulously varied raw vegan food. Huge parts of America are simply not set up for raw vegans.

So set aside the idea of numerous ingredients, spices and tools. They're too cumbersome to travel with; I know—I've tried it. Even if you *could* find space for it all, unless you have a personal valet to pack, set up, then repack everything for you, it's way too much effort.

Not to mention, it can seriously cut into your vacation fun time!

Mix It Up

Abandon the concept that you have to eat meals at specific times and that they have to look a certain way. Know that you'll have good things to eat when you're hungry and let go of everything else. If you think of all your food as delicious "snacks," it tends to take the pressure off preparing entire meals and makes things lighter and simpler. Plus, to me, snacking on raw foods all day ups my travel-foods fun quotient: I'm eating a little differently than I usually do, which feels "vacation-y," but I'm still getting the high-quality ingredients and powerhouse nutrition I love.

Eat the Ingredients, Skip the Dish

The trick here is to eat the *ingredients* without processing them into what you'd typically prepare, like burgers, pastas and calzones, or whatever fabulous raw food you're putting together at home. Focus on consumption of high-quality ingredients. Instead of making and storing an apple pie, for example, bring the apples, nuts/seeds and dates or raisins, and eat these. No refrigeration or fork required!

Eating the whole food makes everything—preparing, packing,

storing and consuming—much, much simpler. It also allows you to combine the various ingredients in a number of different ways. This way of eating also comes in handy when I have a particularly busy week at home as well.

Modify, Simplify and Lower Your Standards (a bit)

And don't beat yourself up about any of it! I'm not talking about going straight for the snack cakes and soda, but if the choice is between non-raw almond butter and going to bed hungry, maybe make an exception. Remember that starving or stressing about your food isn't healthy either. Don't cancel out all the benefits of eating raw vegan by worrying about how you're going to do it.

Food Storage and Utensils on the Road

I'm a woman happily obsessed by containers; I'm pretty sure it all started with those little nesting barrels I played with as a little girl. This trait has served me well when traveling.

Storage methods depend on the length and type of trip, but in general I reuse and adapt a few basic items for my travel adventures. Keep in mind that the ultimate container goal is to compact, nest and/or eliminate lightweight containers as we use them. Below are the tips I've found most useful over the years.

- **Cooler**: If not flying and checking your cooler, use a soft-sided one. A hard one will be just as large when you return home as when you left. At hotels, ask for a small fridge. If there is no freezer/fridge option, you can fill up your cooler daily with ice from the hotel ice machine.

- **Ice packs**: Reusable hard ice packs (which you can fly with) or ice sheets (which are pliable and can be cut to fit any sized cooler, but which may be confiscated by TSA) are both extremely handy. Both will outlast actual ice and won't create a soggy mess at the bottom of your cooler. You can easily refreeze them at your various destinations.

- **Compact, insulated (and foldable) lunchbag**: Use one of these little guys to throw some snacks in for a day trip, on a flight, or while you're away from your main cooler.

- **Reusable grocery sacks**: Pack your dry goods in a reusable, packable grocery bag. I'm a fan of Envirosax and ChicoBag. They last forever, hold a ton, are eco-aware and come in many styles.

- **Individual food containers**: I travel with plastic, BPA-free nesting containers.

- **Beverage containers**: A sports bottle with a lid for mixing greens/protein powders and for taking your liquids with you is a lifesaver. Also, don't forget your filtering water bottle.

- **Utensils:** In a pinch, you can pick up plastic utensils and paper napkins at the airport, hotel or a local fast food joint and carry them in a plastic zip bag. Or even better, pack bamboo or compostable utensils or even just regular flatware and cloth napkins. Remember that if you're flying you'll need to make sure whatever you bring is allowable by TSA guidelines.

Breakfasts for Travel

With these tips in mind, let's get started on the actual *food* you're going to pack on your adventures. Now I realize I suggested letting go of the concept of breakfasts, lunches and dinners. But travel breakfasts are so easy that you can make an exception if you want to. You can certainly get fancy if you've got the time and inclination, but I recommend keeping it simple, at least at the outset.

Having a couple of breakfast options can be nice, but just as often I'll pack a single breakfast to eat every morning for the entire trip. Below are a few of my favorites.

- **Granola and Cereal**: A quick Internet search will result in a plethora of granola recipes, but you don't really need a recipe at all. You can mix up whatever you've got on hand, add some spices and you're good to go. I often use sunflower seeds, cinnamon, pumpkin seeds, Brazil nuts, buckwheat, coconut flakes and raisins. I never measure, but tend to stay heavy on the seeds-to-nuts ratio. I simply toss handfuls of ingredients into the food processor and lightly chop, always stirring in the raisins after I remove my cereal from the processor so they remain whole. I pour this mixture into a plastic bag because it's easy to travel with and gets more compact as you go. (I'm generally not fond of plastic bags, but remember: simplify, modify and lower your standards here. I also reuse plastic bags over and over.)

- **Chia and fruit**: Pack a bag of chia seeds. When you're ready for breakfast, pour out a quarter cup or so, add a cut-up banana, some water (warm water is sometimes nice) and maybe a dash of cinnamon. Voilà! You have one of my favorite breakfasts—one that can be eaten any time of the day.

- **Banana and sunflower seeds:** Though I do recommend soaking, sprouting and dehydrating your own seeds before you go (for the simple reason that purchasing them will cost you an arm and a leg), once you're on the road, it doesn't get much easier than this breakfast option. Just peel the banana, dip into the seeds and go!

- **Raw vegan protein powder/meal replacement powder:** Shake this up with some water in a sports bottle and you're off. You can also add this to your chia cereal for an extra boost.

- **Greens powder**: Shake and go with this as well. I almost always drink greens powder several times a day while traveling. Great nutrition, tasty and easy, easy, easy.

Snacks

As mentioned above, snacks will be the meat of your raw food travel repertoire—*nut* meat, that is!

Remember: what we're really doing here is packing the raw ingredients that we'd normally process into more complex meals and just eating them whole. This way they pack, travel and store easily and efficiently.

I've grouped the snack ideas below by location—where they can be acquired when on the road—as well as by what you can prep and pack at home ahead of time.

Hotel or Airport

Spotting snacks here can be a challenge, but fruit and maybe even some raw nuts or seeds (they won't be soaked, of course) can usually be found in both locations. Prepackaged salads are often readily available as well. Starbucks, for example, is fairly common in airports and locations close to hotels, and can be a good source for some of these items. Organic may not be an option.

Standard Grocery Store

If your only food source is a Safeway or Vons, for example, here are some ideas:

- **Fruit**: Fruits with rinds or peels, like oranges, grapefruits and bananas, travel best. Note: a lot of people will run immediately to the dried fruit section for traveling but seriously, besides raisins in your cereal or a few dates as a sweets fix, my advice is to skip it. Dried fruit is very high in sugar and is murder on your teeth, especially if you're not as diligent about brushing while traveling as you might be at home.

- **Veggie sticks**: Any veggie that can be cut up and eaten raw—including cucumber, zucchini, carrots, celery, summer squash.

- **Cherry/grape tomatoes, grapes**: So easy to pick, pack, store and eat.

- **Avocados**: The humble avocado is one of my favorite travel foods and therefore deserves its own bullet point. It's delicious and comes in its own carrying case (although I will often place it in a container so as not to squish it).

Health-food Store, Co-op or Whole Foods

If you have access to any of these, you're good to go! The following items should be readily available (and of course, if you're able to plan ahead, you can bring them from home):

- **Raw hummus**: This can be scooped up with a spoon or cucumber chips, bell peppers or zucchini chips (simply cut up these goodies and dive right in). Note: If you're flying, hummus is considered a liquid, so either check it or forget it.

- **Raw sauerkraut**: Delicious! A few companies have come out with some downright tantalizing flavor combinations. I eat it straight out of the container.

- **Raw soaked/sprouted seeds and nuts**: While these will cost you, many stores such as Whole Foods sell these in bulk. Smaller packages can also be purchased and are a tasty treat.

- **Guacamole**: Guacamole can serve as a meal in itself, or dip and enjoy with cut up veggies, raw bread or crackers.

- **Garlic spread**: Oh my goodness, do I love garlic spread! This can take an avocado or wrap from yum to *HOLYSMOKESTHAT'SAMAZING!*

- **Raw tahini and nut/seed butters**: These can be a little more costly than some snacks, but they're easy to swipe onto crackers, bread or apple slices. Trader Joe's sometimes carries raw almond butter for a fraction of the usual health-food store cost, but I often order mine online (Artisana brand) in eight-pound tubs from Amazon and allocate to small containers for travel (also considered a liquid and must be checked when flying).

- **Raw bars**: Bars can serve as an easy meal alternative. If you're extra sensitive to sweets, however, skip these as they can be quite high in sugar, particularly if they feature a lot of dried fruit.

- **Crackers/breads**: Some stores may offer raw vegan crackers and breads. These tend to be a bit pricey, but they can be a fun addition to your menu every once in a while. Sometimes you just want some variety!

- **Wraps**: Raw packaged flatbread or coconut wraps are also somewhat pricey, but with avocado and garlic spread they're absolute *heaven*.

- **Nori wrapped seed pâtés**: These tiny wonders are made by Go Pals (official product name: Nori Wrapped Energy Sticks) and are delicious. They come in a variety of flavors, such as Texas BBQ, Italian and Curry. They look a bit like taquitos and taste something like jerky. They don't require refrigeration and are made of raw vegan, sprouted, high-enzyme goodness.

- **Chlorella tablets**: These are terrific for travel. They aid in detoxification and are a highly nutritious superfood boasting over twenty vitamins and minerals that improve digestion and support immune system function. They also help keep your mind sharp—all great benefits to counteract some of the stresses inherent with travel. Make sure to bring your toothbrush, however: chlorella gives you a nice, temporary case of blackish-green witch teeth—perfect for scaring your fellow travelers.

- **Honey sticks**: These are not vegan of course, but if you're open to it and know a supplier where you can obtain raw organic honey from sustainably and kindly-raised bees, honey can be an option. These little straw-like sticks are ideally suited for popping in your purse or backpack.

Prep at Home and Pack

Most of the above items can be prepared at home and packed for a fraction of the packaged-item price. With packaged raw foods, we really pay for convenience. I tend to prepare items that don't require refrigeration, are largely unavailable at my destination or are very expensive on the road and which add variety to my meals. Some of my on-the-road (and at-home) favorites are:

- **Soaked, sprouted and dehydrated nuts and seeds**: Save a bundle by preparing them yourself. Packaged nuts and seeds are often quite salty as well.

- **Sea stix**: The homemade version of the Nori Wrapped Energy Sticks discussed above. A bit tricky to make at first (and mine never look as good as the packaged ones), but easy, fast and tasty.

- **Crackers**: So fast and easy to make at home. As with all dehydrated foods, make sure to dry them completely before packing.

- **Bread sticks**: These dry more quickly in the dehydrator than bread loaves and are fun and easy to pack in individually-sized portions for day hikes and other short trips.

- **Bread**: Making raw bread may seem daunting, but minus soaking, sprouting and dehydrating time, it takes all of about ten minutes. I prepare small loaves for traveling and pack these into a plastic or cloth bag.

- **Protein bars**: When I make these myself I ditch the dried fruit (except for raisins) and use a base of buckwheat and seeds.

- **Soup**: Soup?? Yes, soup! This is one of my favorite suggestions, culled from Sergei and Valya Boutenko's wonderful book, *Fresh: The Ultimate Live-Food Cookbook*. Dehydrate any veggies on hand, add spices and pack into a plastic bag. Simply shake some into a cup or bowl, add hot water, rehydrate and stir. Not quite like the real thing, but still: soup!

Beverages

As mentioned in the section on packing above, a key tip here is to travel with your own filtering water bottle. I find this to be indispensable for providing quality drinking water wherever I go. I will even use filtered water out of my travel bottle to wash my face on the road.

Hotel, Airport or Standard Grocery Store

You will be able to obtain these items at most airports, hotels and standard grocery stores:

- **Water**: Obviously fresh water is available almost anywhere in the U.S., but BEWARE: If potable water is *not* available where you're traveling, rethink and be very cautious about eating raw food while there. While you may be able to purchase safe bottled water for drinking, remember that raw foods need to be washed in potable water as well because they will be consumed without any kind of heat processing that would destroy harmful organisms.

- **Tea bags:** Generally, commercially available tea is not truly raw (although you can dry your own herbs and make your own), but it's nice to have something warm to drink from time to time. Consider also the medicinal value of steeped herbs. While traveling you can carry your favorite tea bags wherever you go and take advantage of the hot water available at hotels and conferences. If you have access to a tea kettle, simply warm the water (dip a finger in to make sure it's not too hot to touch) instead of boiling it.

- **Lemon water**: There is just something luxurious and spa-like about lemon water. Lemons are often available at buffets, salad bars, airports and hotels.

- **Coconut water**: Though not devoid of sugar, coconut water is chock-full of nutrients, such as potassium, calcium, magnesium, phosphorous and sodium, which regulate mineral balance, maintain energy, relax muscles and hydrate. These days, coconut water is available almost everywhere, including many convenience stores.

Health-food Store, Co-op or Whole Foods

You're golden if you've got access to one of these. Plenty of beverages to choose from.

Prep and Pack at Home

Your trusty filtering water bottle will do just fine here. However, I often purchase greens powder, teas and protein powder before my trip so I have my favorite brands and flavors with me on the road.

Desserts

Raw vegan desserts are well known for their high degree of deliciosity. If you've got a sweet tooth, there's no need to leave it at home.

Hotels or Airport

Just as with snacks, your choices are somewhat limited here. But between the hotel/airport mini-stores and local Starbucks or other coffee house, you should be able to find some dried fruit. I know, I said I don't love dried fruit because of the tooth-decay issue. But if you're roaming your hotel halls at night, absolutely jonesing for some sweets, go with the dried fruit.

Standard Grocery Store

Dried fruits again; see above. I like dates in particular. They're a great candy replacement.

Health-food Store, Co-op or Whole Foods

You have no worries if you've got access to some specialty food stores like these. Usually you'll find all kinds of treats, such as:

- **Packaged raw vegan "cheesecake" slices**: Delicious, though not cheap! Often made with nuts.

- **Tarts, cookies, chocolates and macaroons:** All of these can be found in raw form at your local health-food store.

- **Ice cream**: There are some great brands of raw ice cream out there to try on the road. These are generally made with cashews or coconut rather than dairy.

Prep at Home and Pack

Depending on how you feel about preparing foods ahead of time, and how much time and effort you have to put into it, you can prepare any number of your own raw vegan desserts to take on the road. I suggest making bite-sized portions that are easier to pack and eat. Cookies are great companions. Macaroons, for example, are very simple to whip up and travel with. Brownies, lemon bars, tarts, and cheesecake bites are also simple and yummy treats on the road.

Replenishment on the Road

Maybe you're extending your trip or you simply ate *everything* you packed on the train ride over. Not to worry! You can always Google raw vegan restaurants, or check out happycow.net for vegan options (Happy Cow doesn't currently offer "raw" as a search feature but you can definitely make use of the "vegan" option).

You might also be amazed at the specialty health-food stores I've dug up over the years in some out-of-the way places across middle America, using nothing but my phone. Usually these often dusty little shops are owned by a very interesting character who works the register, carries items you'd never in your life expect to find in the middle of nowhere, and is delighted to chat with you about your shared health interests.

Farmers' markets and even convenience stores (you can almost always find a banana and maybe even a packaged salad) are good options to consider too.

Remember: Have Fun!

Raw vegan traveling requires a little thinking ahead, especially for longer trips, but it can yield delightful results, including feeling fantastic and getting the most out of your time away. Whatever happens, remember to *lower your standards* and just do your best. Keeping a spirit of fun while exploring your new surroundings is key to enjoying your adventures.

When visiting Bondi Beach in Australia before a retreat, I happened upon a tiny corner grocery store that sold raw nuts and made fresh veggie juices on the spot. Thank goodness! I was also able to find greens powder in another nearby specialty health food store. This, along with the kind and open-minded retreat chef who allowed me to blend smoothies with his high-powered blender in the kitchen, buoyed me through the rest of the trip. Stay open and experiment and you never know what amazing new food finds you may encounter on your exploits.

Bon voyage!

* Even during the best of times, packing for vacation can be a convoluted affair. To make life just a little bit easier in those moments I've included a Raw Vegan Travel Checklist on the following pages.

Raw Vegan Travel Checklist

Containers and supplies:

- Plastic zip bags
- Nesting, BPA-free plastic food containers
- Soft-sided cooler
- Small lunch tote
- Reusable grocery sack
- Hard ice packs or ice sheets
- Filter bottle
- Sports bottle
- Utensils
- Napkins

Staples:

- Protein powder and/or meal replacement powder
- Greens powder
- Chlorella tablets

Breakfast Options:

- Granola
- Chia
- Bananas (and/or other fruit)

Snacks:

- Veggie sticks
- Fruits
- Cherry tomatoes

- Grapes
- Avocado
- Hummus
- Sauerkraut
- Guacamole
- Garlic spread
- Nut/seed butters
- Protein bars
- Crackers
- Bread/bread sticks
- Energy sticks ("sea stix")
- Honey sticks
- Soaked and dehydrated nuts and seeds

Beverages:

- Tea bags
- Coconut water
- Lemon water

Desserts:

- Dried fruit
- Dates
- Cookies
- Cheesecakes, brownies etc.

Part III

Beyond the Fork:
The Raw Food Lifestyle

Chapter Ten

Raw Lifestyle Basics

B esides eating raw food, what do we mean when we talk about the "raw food lifestyle"? As we saw at the beginning of this book, it's the idea of reconnection with self and the bigger picture. It's about remembering our place in nature and the world.

When we eat raw food we begin to comprehend our connection with Mother Earth and with who we really are. Raw food aids in removing the physical, psychological and emotional junk that disconnects us from our bodies, our hearts and the world. It helps us remember how to listen to our bodies, to rediscover what we like, what we don't like—and how it feels to really be alive.

But we need more than just food to create healthy, connected lives. On a very basic level, we also require exercise, social interaction, connection with nature, meaningful work/play (the difference lies only in perception) and good sleep. We also need to alternate between activities by listening to ourselves and responding to our needs moment by moment.

Exercise

Our bodies were designed to move. Although we often compare them to machines or computers, they're infinitely more complex and alive than that. As a general rule, our bodies become better, stronger and more efficient with use. When we sit in an office chair all day, every day, it's going to negatively affect us; our bodies were built for movement. A sedentary lifestyle is an enormous health risk factor. Getting at least thirty minutes of brisk physical activity a day (and integrating movement throughout your day), will go a long way towards supporting overall health.

So let's get moving!

Building exercise into your life on a daily basis doesn't have to mean heading to the gym every day, although if you enjoy that, you certainly can. But remember: even if you're a gym rat, a one- or two-hour workout can't counteract the effects of sitting in an office chair for eight hours! Movement must be incorporated into your whole life.

Ultimately, you want to become so in tune with yourself that you simply respond to your needs as they arise. Most of us need to gradually come back into connection, however, after years (or even a lifetime) of ignoring our needs.

Finding ways to reintegrate movement into your day may take a bit of creativity at first, but here are some ideas:

- Set the alarm on your phone for every hour or—even better—every half hour. Stand up, stretch and take a brisk walk to get a drink of water or just take a lap around the room or office. Whether you're working from home or in an office, I highly recommend this little book for some fun and useful ideas: *Office Yoga: Simple Stretches for Busy People* by Darrin Zeer.

- Replace your desk chair with an exercise ball of the correct height (making sure your knees, elbows and chin are at 90 degree angles while working). This helps to build core muscles and can be a godsend to those with lower back pain.

- Attend a class: yoga, CrossFit, Zumba or Pilates—anything that will get you moving.

- Join (or go to) the gym: I love the gym; it feels like my home away from home. I go three times a week and alternate strength training with cardio work on my off-gym days.

- Walking is the exercise our bodies were designed for. Walk through your neighborhood in the morning, at night and during the workday if you can. If you have dogs and live in an apartment, walking probably isn't a choice but a requirement! I've walked my dogs for years and even though sometimes it's the *last* thing I actually want to do, it gets me out of the house and into a little bit of nature. Our brisk walks get my blood moving and I get to spend a half hour or more with my pups! Win, win, win, win!

- Bike, rollerblade (that still exists, right?), skateboard or fly a kite! What can you do that sounds fun and gets you out and about?

- If team sports are your thing, join some kind of league. This can be a great social outlet and it also provides accountability for actually showing up! I've even tried a badminton Meetup group!

Everyone knows what exercise means. Just get up and do it! Start where you are, build up, and don't forget to stretch! My daily routine includes stretching every morning and it makes a HUGE difference in my day.

Social Interaction

We are all wired, to one degree or another, for social interaction. Making sure we connect with each other and our community is part of a healthy lifestyle. For my own part, I'm a bit of a loner and have been known to spend three days working from home with my dogs, perfectly content without any human interaction. But after three days, I start getting cabin fever and can begin feeling a little depressed.

Healthy social interaction means different things to different folks, depending on what your daily life is like. Obviously if you're married with kids, your social needs will be different than if you live alone. In the latter case you may need to put a little more effort into connecting with others.

Connection with Nature

We've already talked about how simply eating raw food reconnects you with nature. When you're eating whole foods, you interact with the actual plant. This rarely fails to bring me to a place of gratitude. While plants are not necessarily sentient beings in the same way that animals are, they certainly are alive and respond to stimuli. Before I juice or make food, I like to place my hands on the food, feel its energy and offer gratitude for it—for the plant that is about to merge its life energy with mine.

Having said this, in addition to eating raw food we also need to spend time in nature to be in optimal health. Dr. Richard Louv, in *Last Child in the Woods,* identifies a syndrome called Nature Deficit Disorder. When our lives are bereft of nature, we can experience symptoms including attention disorders, depression, mood disorders and increased perception of stress.

Psychologist Dr. Rachel Kaplan of the University of Michigan found that "office workers with a view of nature liked their jobs more, enjoyed better health and reported greater life satisfaction."[64]

Roger S. Ulrich, Ph.D., Director of the Center for Health Systems and Design at Texas A&M University, discovered that nature can help the body heal. Ulrich analyzed the effect that window views had on patients recovering from abdominal surgery. He found that:

> Patients whose hospital rooms overlooked trees had an easier time recovering than those whose rooms overlooked brick walls. Patients able to see nature got out of the hospital faster, had fewer complications and required less pain medication than those forced to stare at a wall.[65]

Consider incorporating the following activities into your daily routine to reconnect with nature:

- Get outside! Take a walk and notice nature all around you. Make regular trips to parks or take hikes.

- Go camping!

- Purchase houseplants—and take care of them!

- Plant an herb garden, either indoors (on a windowsill) or outside.

- Plant trees and plants where you'll be able to see them outside your windows.

- Bring plants to your office. Place a plant on your desk.

- Discover your area's botanical gardens, rose gardens, etc.

Meaningful Work/Play

Alan Watts said, "This is the real secret of life—to be completely engaged with what you are doing in the here and now. And instead of calling it work, realize it is play." Creating space in life for rewarding work and play is essential. Notice that defining something as either "work" or "play" can simply be a matter of perspective. What is play for me may be work for you, and vice versa. However, engaging in activities that are meaningful to you, for whatever reason, and feeling purpose in what you do can be immensely satisfying. If you're not sure what this means for you, I humbly refer you to my book, *Guided by Your Own Stars: Connect with the Inner Voice and Discover Your Dreams.* In that book I take you from disconnected to full connection through easy exercises and experiments anyone can complete.

Many people think finding rewarding work means quitting their current job and fulfilling a long-time dream. It's true that doing what inspires you is wildly important. Even so, finding joy and fulfillment in what you're doing at the moment has more to do with who you're *being* while you're doing it, right here, right now. This relates to self-connection and the ability to dwell in the present moment. Offering your full presence to a task—whether it's paperwork, tending to a sick animal or anything else—opens up time and allows you to fully engage with the activity. This is the experience of *flow.*

I'm not going to go deeply into the idea of flow here, but everyone knows the experience: you're engaged in an activity and the next thing you know an hour has flown by—you've been fully present in what you were doing. For a detailed study of flow, check out Mihaly Csikszentmihalyi's book *Flow: The Psychology of Optimal Experience.*

The following activities may help kick-start flow in your daily experience:

- Meditation: there's nothing like meditation to reconnect you with who you really are and help you slow down and practice presence.

- Take time to breathe during the day! Attention on the breath can be a trusted ally in returning awareness to the present moment.

- Explore interests that may be new or almost forgotten: if you love animals, for example, consider volunteering in a shelter or rescue, walking a neighbor's dog or checking to see if any of your skills could be of use for a local non-profit.

- Try a sport, a dance class or other physical activity. Keeping the attention out of the mind and on the body is key!

- Experiment with bringing absolute presence into tasks (especially those you find boring) at work or home. Notice that it is impossible to be bored while engaging your attention fully; boredom is really just an abstract judgment.

- Talk to others who are experiencing flow in their lives and engaging in work they find rewarding. See what their experience is and explore whether you can find any corollaries in your own life.

Quality Sleep

Sleep is one of my favorite activities! Waking up well rested, detoxed and refreshed is something I absolutely love. There is no way to experience life at full capacity without the rejuvenating benefits of sleeping well. Our bodies need sleep to recover, detox and rebuild.

Most of us need between seven and nine hours per night. While many people survive on much less, not prioritizing sleep is asking for trouble.

Not getting enough sleep over long periods of time increases the risk of many diseases and psychiatric problems and disconnects us from our true capacity to experience life fully. Even short-term sleep deprivation can result in issues with cognition (memory, concentration), anxiety, weight gain (hunger hormones are easily disrupted by lack of sleep), distractibility, and impaired task performance.

I've found that not using electric lights or screens after dark most of the time (I do use candles) and rising and setting with the sun when possible improves my quality of sleep tremendously and helps me feel fantastic. This practice also reconnects me with the Earth's cycles, which all of us are wired around whether we know it or not.

Check out the following ideas for getting great sleep:

- Create a sleep routine to help you get into the "sleep zone," including rising and retiring at approximately the same time each day. Our bodies prefer routines, and having one for bedtime will greatly improve your chances of getting to sleep when you're ready. This can include meditating, lighting a candle, taking a shower or bath, etc. Whatever makes you feel calm and allows your body to wind down.

- Stay off of computer and phone screens and switch off the television a couple hours before bedtime. The blue light emitted from screens prevents the brain from secreting melatonin, which helps us fall and stay soundly asleep. If you absolutely MUST be on a screen, download f.lux or a similar app to decrease exposure to blue light. You can also don some super sexy orange-lens glasses.

- Make a to-do list prior to going to bed. Get those tasks out of your brain and on to paper.

- Avoid caffeine, alcohol, sugar and other substances that interfere with sleep patterns and quality.

- Engage in regular exercise. Taking a brisk walk in the evenings can be part of a healthy pre-sleep routine, as it can aid in relaxation and reduce anxiety.

- Make sure you get some light exposure in the morning and early in the day. This is thought to assist in normalizing sleep patterns.

- Use black-out curtains. It's important to have your sleeping area as dark as possible. Cover lights (I throw a sweatshirt over my air purifier's "on" light) and use a sleep mask if necessary. Pay attention to light pollution in your sleeping area, such as from streetlights or other light sources.

- Eat your last meal of the day a couple of hours prior to going to bed. Eating lightly before sleeping allows the body to spend its rest time recovering, detoxing and rebuilding rather than digesting. I feel much better in the morning when I simply drink a smoothie or have a light meal in the evenings.

- Use a little lavender essential oil on your pillow. Research shows that lavender eases anxiety and insomnia.

♥   ♥   ♥

Creating space for self-care, including exercise, social interaction, time in nature, meaningful work/play and good quality sleep will benefit anyone and everyone. But as you delve into the raw food lifestyle and become more and more sensitive to the needs of your body and to your connection with nature, this reconnecting time is absolutely essential for optimal health and a fantastic, fulfilled life experience.

Chapter Eleven

Health Care

Periodic medical testing to track your health is just a flat-out good idea. And if you decide to transition to raw vegan foods, visits with a qualified health care practitioner can provide peace of mind. You'll know you're monitoring what you need to be monitoring and looking out for potential pitfalls.

That said, it may be a challenge to partner with a practitioner who truly understands and supports your decision to eat raw. While we tend to think of doctors as *health* specialists, they are often *disease* specialists instead.

I'll borrow a quote from a Heidi Klum hair product commercial and say that in my opinion, treating disease rather than preventing it through healthy food and lifestyle choices is "working at the wrong end of hair."

We will always want access to acute care in the case of emergencies or injuries, such as broken bones. But a professional who explores the more subtle aspects of health, healing and preventive care, including an emphasis on the causes of symptoms and not just how to suppress them, is worth his or her weight in gold.

Thankfully, progressive professionals with backgrounds in wellness are popping up with increasing frequency. It may take some effort, but keep at it; they're out there, and many of the "new guard" physicians are more open to alternative perspectives. With the help of the Internet and word of mouth, you're sure to find someone who's a good fit for you.

Choosing a Health Care Professional

Your ideal practitioner will be someone with whom you feel comfortable going to for checkups and health maintenance issues. Beyond that, selecting which medical/health professionals to engage with is a personal choice. You will have you own reasons for consulting a practitioner, as well as your own preferences, so I've necessarily kept this chapter short and to the essentials. The main takeaway is that whenever you make a major shift in your diet or lifestyle, it's a good idea to find a practitioner to support you on your new path.

In my own case, for years my employer provided my medical insurance. Two options were offered. Both were large groups that were all but useless to me, although I did take advantage of covered periodic medical testing as recommended by my naturopathic doctor. In general, I opted to pay out-of-pocket for alternative services I felt were more in line with supporting true health and wellness for me. I was also fortunate to find a naturopathic physician I liked. Over the years I've benefited from additional specialties, including acupuncture, acupressure, holistic chiropractic services, herbalists, massage, dermatology and hypnotherapy. Through research and word of mouth, I've been able to locate many wonderful professionals who provide integrated and holistic services.

Currently I pay for my own insurance simply to retain access to acute care should there be an emergency, but other than for lab work and an occasional work-related physical, I generally don't use it. I continue to pay out-of-pocket for my alternative services; these are my health-maintenance professionals. Fortunately options for coverage of these "alternative" services that actually support ongoing optimal health are becoming somewhat more common with some insurance, so check your policy.

Tips for Locating Health Professionals

Get Clear on What You're Looking For

Do you want to try an alternative therapist such as an acupuncturist, or would you prefer a physician who will monitor blood work or keep an eye on your overall health? Both can be quite useful and are by no means mutually exclusive.

Word of Mouth

My favorite method of referral is through people I know and trust. Send out a Facebook post, tweet or take advantage of friends' knowledge or other social media access points and request ideas from those in your area.

Professional Referrals

Discuss preferred providers with nutritionists, chiropractors and other alternative health professionals you already trust. Health care practitioners often consult with each other so they can offer a treasure trove of information regarding physicians who may be open to alternative treatments, diets and lifestyles.

Check Credentials

If you're looking for a physician, be certain that they actually have a medical or naturopathic degree—or whatever type of degree they *should* have. It can vary with the profession. A chiropractor is a D.C., a naturopath is an N.D., and so on. But there are many certification programs that may sound "doctor-y" but which do not actually offer accredited medical degrees, so be aware of what you're looking for and do a little extra research as needed.

Make an Appointment

If it feels right, make an appointment. Ask if you can schedule an initial consultation to see if you and the practitioner will be a good fit for each other. Some professionals offer an initial consultation at no cost.

Don't Be Afraid to Move On

Remember to treat your health like the gift it is. Don't worry about hurting a practitioner's feeling if they're not a good fit for you for one reason or another. If you feel they are trustworthy, perhaps they can make a recommendation for a more appropriate referral. The important thing is to find a professional with whom you feel comfortable to have on hand as you embark on your journey.

Chapter Twelve

Basic Nutrition and Supplementation

As human animals we need to ingest a variety of micronutrients and macronutrients. The former include vitamins and minerals, antioxidants and enzymes, while macronutrients are the body's main sources of energy: proteins (amino acids), fats and carbohydrates. We also require fiber (found in carbohydrates) and water to stay healthy. The varied organic raw vegan food diet provides all of these in spades. Still, some people feel supplementation is beneficial. While alternating your sources of nutrients is extremely important, in some situations we are not able to obtain a wide enough variety or sufficient quality of nutrients. In others situations we may want to target a specific issue. Either way, supplementation, whether in pill form or liquid formulation and via vitamins, "superherbs" or "superfoods,"[66] can significantly upgrade our nutritional profile.

Depending on diet and personal physical makeup, raw foodists *can* be vulnerable to deficiencies of B12 and omega-3 essential fatty acids. We'll discuss ways to get these into your diet below.

Foods in their natural state provide the exact nutrients we need; our food evolved with us, and vice versa. As raw vegans, by not destroying those nutrients with cooking or otherwise highly processing our food, we're in the best position to be getting the best nutrition. If we're eating a quality, seasonal, varied diet composed mainly of raw organic leafy greens and other vegetables, fruit, nuts and seeds, we're on the right track for ideal nutrition.

In this chapter, I briefly address vitamin and mineral supplements from a raw food perspective. We also revisit the topics of protein, fat, carbohydrates and fiber, and explore a few supplemental items and superfoods you can consider adding to your raw food repertoire. Many of these topics are quite complex, and we'll only touch on them here; I suggest exploring further on your own and with your network of health care providers.

Vitamin and Mineral Supplements

A vitamin is an organic compound (nutrient) needed for proper physical functioning that cannot be synthesized in adequate amounts by the body. There are thirteen classified vitamins, which are grouped into water soluble (B vitamins and vitamin C) and fat soluble (A, D, E and K) vitamins, depending on how the vitamin is absorbed, stored and excreted. Most vitamins are obtained from food (often via bacterial action), although a few are manufactured by gut flora (K and B7, which is biotin) and as we'll discuss below, B12 is processed by soil organisms. One form of vitamin D is synthesized through the skin via sunlight. Some vitamins can also be produced by the body using precursors.

Dietary minerals are chemical elements needed for physical functioning. For mammals, these include (in order of most required to least): calcium, phosphorus, potassium, sulfur, sodium chlorine, and magnesium. Known trace minerals needed for life functions are iron, cobalt, copper, zinc, manganese, molybdenum, iodine, bromine and selenium. Not all of the elements needed for life are known. Most elements are absorbed by plants through the soil (we depend on bacteria to process many of them), and move up the food chain. This is one reason why soil health is so important.

As noted, as raw vegans, we're in a great position to be getting a wide variety of vitamins and minerals as we're not destroying them by cooking and heavy processing.

Why Supplement?

Everyone seems to hold their own opinions about supplementation. These run the gamut from the belief that supplements are a waste of money (and even harmful), to the other extreme—the belief that one cannot be healthy *without* supplements.

One argument against supplementation is the issue of the ingredients, quality and regulation of supplements themselves. Technically, supplements are regulated by the FDA, but only as "special food substances"—not as medications. This basically means that they are considered safe until proven otherwise. No analysis or checking is performed unless a significant problem arises.

Hence, supplement companies operate on the honor system, and not always to great effect. Multiple studies have found that an alarming number of randomly tested supplements did not contain what was on the label at all, and some actually contained harmful substances. Efforts to provide safe and accurately labeled supplements are being driven from within the supplement industry at this time. These include voluntary testing and a certification or seal-of-approval process. Though analyses vary from lab to lab, currently, third-party, independent supplement "seals of approval" are awarded from:

- Consumerlab.com

- The U.S. Pharmacopeial Convention (USP)

- NSF International

A second argument against supplements is the idea that you can get all the nutrients you need from a balanced diet. This may have been true once upon a time; soil was in good condition,[67] our food was not overly processed and high-quality food was readily available and a part of everyone's diet. Nowadays all sorts of factors—soil quality, farming practices, freezing, transportation, storage and so on—can negatively impact the nutritional value of even the healthiest foods. You may also remember from Chapter Two, Dr. Howard Jacobson's observations on how variable the nutritional content of even healthy food can be.

This means that although raw vegans are getting more nutrients than those on a Standard American Diet, even raw fooders could arguably benefit from considering supplementation to fill in any nutritional gaps.

While I'm not an expert in this area, I can offer advice in keeping with the theme of this book: there is no substitute for listening to our bodies and getting as much of our nutritional needs met via actual foods. Consulting health professionals you trust is also recommended.

I personally feel comfortable taking a high quality, whole foods general supplement, although I do take breaks from it periodically. At the same time, I do not think taking a supplement is absolutely necessary for health if you're eating a varied, organic diet, juicing (a great way to get a concentrated dose of vitamins and minerals) and supplementing using superfoods and herbs. But when I do take one, I prefer a raw vegan whole food supplement for the same reasons I prefer raw vegan whole food. The ingredients, though certainly not in their whole, natural forms, are not heat processed and do not include animal products.

There are several brands of raw supplements out there and I don't recommend one over the other beyond making sure that they are made from whole, raw, vegan, organic foods and do not include harmful excipients (product stabilizers, binders, preservatives, artificial flavors and fillers) that may cause issues. Excipients may include but are not limited to the following:

- Hydrogenated and partially hydrogenated oils: linked to heart problems and strokes.[68]

- Silica: shown to cause autoimmune dysfunction.[69]

- Artificial colors: linked to cancer and hyperactivity.[70]

- Parabens: preservative agents that can cause hormone disruption.[71]

- Lactose: can cause digestive issues in lactose-sensitive individuals.

- Monosodium glutamate (MSG): a proven neurotoxin.[72]

- Talc: linked to cancer.[73]

- Gelatin: derived from animal skin and bones, tendons and ligaments.

- Magnesium stearate: used as a lubricant. Linked to suppressed immune system functioning.[74]

- Titanium dioxide: used as a pigment, can increase inflammatory responses in certain individuals.[75]

A third-party vetted supplement would be ideal to ensure you're ingesting what the label says you are. After all, your supplements are supposed to *help* you, not add to the challenge of keeping your body healthy and getting it the nutrition it needs.

A note on "superfoods": "Superfoods" is a marketing term. It's used to denote foods with high nutritional value. It's important to remember that even if they aren't labeled, these are foods we will be eating all the time on the raw vegan diet (e.g., berries, dark greens, chia, hemp etc.). Regularly eating these foods that are dense in nutrients and that some consider supplemental, is part of what makes eating raw vegan so rejuvenating.

Special Note Regarding B12 for Raw Vegans

Most raw vegans who consume enough calories (which is key!) are getting enough vitamins and minerals, including B12. This is because B12 is actually present in soil and processed by bacteria, which thrive on pre-biotics (e.g., fiber)—which raw vegans get a ton of. If you're eating fruits and veggies from the farm or from your own garden, B12 should definitely be present.

The Framingham study[76] demonstrated that meat eaters are just as likely to be deficient in B12, so this is not really a vegan or raw vegan issue; it's something for everyone to consider. I think it's reasonable to be cautious about B12, as deficiencies can result in permanent neurological damage, and a very small proportion of people have a difficult time absorbing B12 from food sources.

Though there has been some controversy over the bioavailability of plant-based B12, it is possible to obtain B12 from plant-based sources. Fermented foods like miso, for example, can be high in B12. Nutritional yeast, a deactivated yeast that is not technically raw, is something I include regularly in my diet. It is a complete protein and is also often fortified with B12.

My opinion is that it's not worth the risk to NOT supplement B12. It's worth noting that as B12 is a water-soluble vitamin there is little risk of oversupplement. But as previously mentioned, it's good to check B12 levels periodically.

Protein, Amino Acids, and Protein Powders

Let's quickly revisit what protein is. Proteins are molecules comprised of amino acids linked together. Amino acids are organic compounds that are considered building blocks essential for bodily functions in mammals. There are twenty amino acids. Essential amino acids are those that the body cannot synthesize independently. There are generally thought to be eight of these—but these numbers depend on the classification system that is used. These essential amino acids must be derived from our diet.

Proteins derived from plant sources have been found to be superior to animal-based proteins for human consumption. Dr. T. Colin Campbell, in *The China Study,* stated that "There is a mountain of compelling research showing that plant protein allows for slow but steady synthesis of new proteins, and is the healthiest type of protein."[77] Animal-based proteins are associated with a number of diseases and disorders, including promotion of cancer growth, adult-onset diabetes, coronary artery disease and hypertension. Plant-based proteins are not associated with promotion of disease.

It used to be thought necessary to combine foods to provide complete proteins (proteins containing all essential amino acids). This is now known to be a myth. The body keeps a store of amino acids, and provides these perfect protein combinations for us. Jeff Novick, M.S., R.D., and former Director at the Pritikin Center, notes that ". . . you will find that any single whole natural plant food, or any combination of them, if eaten as one's sole source of calories for a day, would provide all of the essential amino acids and not just the *minimum* requirements but far more than the *recommended* requirements. Modern researchers know that it is virtually impossible to design a calorie-sufficient diet based on unprocessed whole natural plant foods that is deficient in any of the amino acids. (The only possible exception could be a diet based solely on fruit)."[78]

That's excellent news for those of us eating tons of unprocessed, whole, natural plant foods!

Though recommendations will vary depending on the source of your data, most agree that humans require protein to make up roughly 5–10 percent of our diets. All whole foods contain protein, with fruit containing approximately 4–8 percent protein and veggies containing even higher protein levels at approximately 10–50 percent. Nuts and seeds also, of course, contain varying amounts of protein. In other words, getting all of your protein needs met through a varied and healthy raw vegan diet isn't an issue.

So while protein powder can serve a purpose in some

situations, I certainly do not think of it as a necessary part of the raw vegan diet. However, I do find protein powder especially useful while traveling, particularly when I'm visiting places I know tend to be weak on the organic produce end.

If you choose to include protein powder in your diet, a variety of raw vegan options exist, including hemp, rice, pea and more. Amino acid supplements are also readily available. As with anything else, carefully read the ingredients on all supplements, and be on the lookout for allergens, fillers and added sugar. If it doesn't say "raw" on the packaging, it's most likely not.

Greens Powders

Greens powders are considered highly nutritious superfoods. But even though they provide concentrated doses of greens, they don't take the place of eating fresh greens! Whole greens are nutritionally balanced. Powders don't guarantee a full array of nutrients, although they do boast antioxidant powers and can be a big help if you've got limited access to a variety of real-live greens.

As with protein powders, I find greens powders quite useful for traveling. In a pinch I'll use them in my smoothies to ensure I'm getting a variety of nutrients if I'm low on whole greens.

Depending on the brand and formulation, you may find any number of ingredients and combinations, including: wheat grass, barley grass, aloe vera, alfalfa, chlorella, spirulina and flax, to name a few. Powders may also include healthy herbs and other substances.

Again, if you're eating enough whole greens, I feel you don't really need greens powders. But if you do want to try one, Sunwarrior is a personal favorite. Everything I noted in the last paragraph about protein powders also applies to greens powders—check the ingredient list to make sure you're getting high quality, organic material without unnecessary ingredients. This is another product that, while not absolutely necessary, can provide a supplemental boost.

Fats and Fatty Acids

Fats are compounds comprised of fatty acid chains. Fatty acids are essentially chains of molecules of varying length, which is why they are categorized into short chain fatty acids (SCFA), medium chain fatty acids (MCFA), long chain fatty acids (LCFA) and very long chain fatty acids (VLCFA). Essential fatty acids are required by the body but cannot be synthesized by it; we must get these from our diet.

There are three general types of dietary fats (the body also makes its own fat from excess calories, but the fat we consume in our diets is referred to as dietary fat):

1. Saturated fats: solid at room temperature, derived mainly from animal sources and implicated in many dietary diseases.

2. Trans fats: most trans fats are created through a food processing method known as partial hydrogenation; they are also implicated in disease and were required to be removed by food companies by 2020.

3. Unsaturated fats: liquid at room temperature. These include monounsaturated fats (found in many foods and oils, generally found to be a positive health ally) and polyunsaturated fats (found primarily in plant foods and considered to be another health ally).

Healthy fats are crucial to physical functioning, forming cell membranes and supplying us with energy. Fats are also converted into other substances needed in our bodies (e.g., hormones). Fatty acids come from animal and plant fats and oils and are categorized into saturated and unsaturated types, depending on the chemical bond.

For human beings, there are only two essential fatty acids: alpha-Linolenic acid or ALA (an omega-3 fatty acid) and LA, or linoleic acid (an omega-6 fatty acid). Most people get a lot of omega-

6 and not enough omega-3 (the ideal ratio is 1:1, and most people on a standard diet are consuming 15:1 or more). The imbalance in this ratio promotes inflammation, and hence encourages a host of diseases, including heart disease, hypertension and diabetes.

Omega-3 fatty acids are categorized into EPA, DHA and ALA. ALA is a precursor to both EPA (eicosapentaenoic acid) and DHA (docosahexaenoic acid). ALA, EPA and DHA, like all so-called essential nutrients, are not produced in significant quantities in the body, and must be derived from diet.

Currently, there is quite a controversy over how to ensure you get enough omega-3 in your diet. Many people advocate animal sources such as fish or krill oil. However, because these are sourced from the ocean there are potential contamination issues (e.g., heavy metals like mercury). Some algae supplements can have similar issues.

On a raw food vegan diet, we can get omega-3 from many sources, including: chia seeds, flax seeds/meal, radish seeds, walnuts, garlic, hemp seeds, fresh basil, oregano, cloves, dried marjoram, broccoli and spinach. I try to eat a good variety of these.

Even with consuming a lot of these foods, I have a difficult time getting (or perhaps absorbing) enough omegas without supplementing using a liquid form. Without this supplement, I sometimes develop very dry hands and feet and get painful little splits in the skin of my fingers and heels.

This is, in fact, the *only* negative health issue I've run into since I've been eating raw food exclusively, and it was easily solved. When I first noticed it I tried a million and one remedies until I finally hit on the actual problem: not enough omega-3. I started taking one tablespoon of Udo's 3-6-9 oil[79] in the morning and one in the evening, and I now have no more issues with this.

In any case, I would certainly take it over the heart disease, stroke and the plethora of other health problems associated with the Standard American Diet!

Carbohydrates & Fiber

The term "carbohydrate" refers to a group of organic compounds that includes sugars, starches and fiber. Carbohydrates are the body's main source of energy, and they are not in short supply. They are found in all whole foods. Carbohydrates are classified as either simple or complex depending on chemical structure and how the body processes them. Simple carbs contain only one or two sugars and are found in foods such as table sugar, fructose (fruit sugar) or dairy sugar (lactose). These are generally absorbed quickly. Complex carbohydrates contain three or more sugars and are often thought of as starchy foods; these are absorbed more slowly. Examples include peanuts, potatoes and corn.

All carbs provide energy, but simple carbohydrates result in bursts of energy that can sometimes cause sugar spikes, while longer-burning, complex carbs can provide sustained energy over a greater period of time.

Generally, whole fruits will not cause a spike in blood sugar like processed sugars will, because the fiber in fruit slows the absorption of the sugars. As we've already seen elsewhere, fiber is essential to digestion and for detoxing out gunk we don't want. This in turn decreases the risk of diseases such as coronary heart disease and diabetes. Fiber is found in whole grains, legumes, fruits and vegetables.

For someone subsisting on the Standard American Diet, fiber supplements might be something to consider. As raw foodies, we automatically get lots of great carbs and fiber!

♥   ♥   ♥

In terms of optimal health, your foundation is made up of your daily raw organic vegan diet, sleep, meaningful work, social interactions, your relationship with nature, and exercise. With raw food, we are getting optimal sources of macronutrients and micronutrients. I personally don't try to keep track of all of them, but I do pay specific attention to areas that are likely deficient in all of us no matter what diet we eat, mainly omega-3s and B12. Our bodies are amazing organisms whose inherent knowledge of nutrition far outstrips current medical science's understanding. Tuning in to the body's signals and noticing how we feel will be our truest compass to health.

Targeting specific issues and bringing about re-regulation and balance can require or at least benefit from supplementation. I mentioned my own case of dry skin and omega-3s, and I've also targeted PMS symptoms using supplementation (I prefer to use superfoods and superherbs, but have also used other supplements).

Supplementation in any form is really a matter of semantics: it really depends on what you're consuming (and *not* consuming) on a regular basis that determines the need or benefit, if any, of consuming additional substances. As with everything else we discuss in this book, I recommend using your best judgement, which will come more from your body than your brain. How do you feel? Do you notice any differences when supplementing with this or that? Is there a specific issue you'd like to target?

As always, pay attention, play it by ear and consult the experts, all the while staying in close connection with your best friend and ally: your own body.

Chapter Thirteen

Raw Pregnancy: A Few Notes on My Experience of Eating for Two!

During the writing of this book, I unexpectedly and joyfully fell in love with the most wonderful man, became engaged and then got pregnant! While we had hoped for a baby from the start, I initially warned my partner that at forty-seven I wasn't sure if pregnancy would realistically be in the cards for us. We decided we were okay with either outcome and, lo and behold, three weeks after officially deciding to start "trying" we were expecting!

Now, while I can't *prove* that being raw vegan impacted my ability to become effortlessly and immediately pregnant at forty-seven years of age, I *can* say that my body was functioning beautifully. My cycles were like clockwork (which they *never* were when I was eating a Standard American Diet), I was in stellar physical condition, and it took no time at all to become pregnant—despite the bleak prediction of only a .06 percent to 5 percent chance of this occurring at all (depending on which source you consult).

Although I dealt with nausea during the first trimester, I

experienced no instances of morning sickness. This despite tossing my cookies two to three times per day for months when pregnant with my son twenty-eight years earlier. Throughout the most recent pregnancy, I had zero major health concerns and generally sailed through with only normal minor backaches and fatigue. I can't say that I noticed either of these being significantly more impactful than when I was eighteen and pregnant with my son.

When I became pregnant this time around, I was eating nearly 100 percent raw vegan, as described in this book. Though I did process some initially challenging thoughts and emotions about letting go of my finely-tuned diet, I was ultimately open to going with any food cravings I experienced during pregnancy, cooked or not. I was ready to accept them as indications that my body needed this or that nutrient. My food choices over the years evolved to an in-tuneness with my body, and I was determined to keep in connection with this knowing and to respect what my system told me it needed. I know how wise and true a friend this body is, and it did not let me down.

During the first trimester I was, like a lot of moms, often nauseous and starving at the same time, and *nothing* sounded good to eat. I could sometimes only choke down fruit, cereal or a banana with almond butter or tahini on it, depending on the day. Several times, out of desperation and fear that I wasn't getting enough nutrients or calories, I ate a cooked item that didn't sound incredibly awful, such as jack-fruit tacos, scrambled or hard-boiled eggs or organic spinach tamales. Not raw or necessarily even vegan selections (in the case of eggs), but not the worst choices either. That was a bit of a rough time, to be sure, but I continued to put on appropriate weight and the pregnancy progressed normally.

To my surprise, however, after getting through the first trimester, I primarily experienced only two cooked-food cravings: eggs and roasted potatoes. (I did eat those organic jack-fruit tacos several times as well—yum!) These cravings happened only periodically. When I ate these I found that my body seemed to deal with them without much difficulty, provided I didn't eat too much. When I did overindulge on a few occasions I felt terrible, slept poorly, and suffered fairly severe food coma and short-term inflammation in my back and joints.

So I did the best I could, and when these cooked-food cravings hit, I ate exclusively organic items in which only high-quality ingredients were used, whether eating out or preparing items myself. I trusted my body, interpreted that it needed something in these foods, and let it go.

I think it's important to note that in addition to first combining households with my partner, when I was pregnant we also moved to a new city. I found myself settling into new routines in a new location, which involved more frequent dining out than normal. This took a bit of getting used to, though my partner was endlessly patient; he took me to the few restaurants and stores that carried the raw food items I was willing to eat, or ran out at a moment's notice to get me whatever food sounded amazing (or merely edible).

With all the moving, unpacking, and changes in routine, it took some time for me to get back up and running with juicing, making smoothies and creating raw food dishes after both moves. By the third trimester I was pretty much back to making these items on a regular basis.

Oftentimes during the pregnancy I made do with fresh, commercially available juices and precut/premade raw food. I had a lot of adjusting to do in a new city, a new home, a new life and in many ways, a new *body*—and although these places were not quite up to my standards of homemade nutrition, they made it much easier to make the necessary adjustments gradually and in a healthy way, for which I'm eternally grateful. I'm fortunate to live in California where I have fairly easy access to all of this goodness.

So by the third trimester, I was essentially back to eating how I'd eaten pre-pregnancy, happily enjoying near-daily green juices and smoothies along with a variety of raw dishes. While pregnant, my body generally craved more higher fat, higher carb and higher protein raw foods than I'd been used to. It also required—in no uncertain terms—MORE of *everything* and *RIGHT NOW*, thank you very much.

One interesting fact was that while I anticipated, feared and braced for lots of "What the hell are you doing??" responses from prenatal healthcare providers regarding my raw vegan diet, this did not happen *even once.* My healthcare team was not only happy with, but impressed by and extremely respectful of my raw vegan food choices. That said, I have to add the weird (or not-so-weird) caveat that my standard Western physicians did not even once *ask* me about my diet (sigh). My midwife inquired, listened to what I ate and then waved an experienced hand at me, saying it was perfect and that there was nothing more she could advise about my nutrition. The same went for my prenatal chiropractor, doula and prenatal massage therapist.

With thirteen weeks to go in the pregnancy, my partner and I enrolled in a twelve-week birthing class, which we dropped out of after only two sessions. During the "nutrition" lecture, we discovered class materials providing the protein content for Fritos, Doritos and hot dogs and recommending a diet that included, fish, dairy, liver and grains! Much of the nutrition information presented was outdated.

Needless to say, this was not a good fit for us. We high-tailed it back to our midwife who laughed with us and offered some excellent books on pregnancy and birthing. She noted too that I did not need anyone to tell me what to eat or how to give birth; the body knows what to do if we know how to tune into it—and boy, do I! My partner was also incredible at reminding me, when I forgot, that I'm very much *guided by my own stars.*

Our checkups and diagnostic scans of our lively new little one relayed perfect results. Vivien was born at home, and she is absolutely the healthiest she could be. Everyone comments on her awareness of all that is going on around her, and she is incredibly socially engaged and engaging. We are so besotted with her! I'm eternally grateful that I knew what my body needed during pregnancy. I have no regrets or questions about what I consumed during her prenatal development. I know I provided her with the best food the planet has to offer.

One caveat. Please remember what I've said throughout this book: it's important that you talk with a trusted medical professional about your diet. This is even more true when you're eating for two! I wanted to share my personal experience in the hopes that it would be interesting and provide additional information about the raw food diet. BUT: proper nutrition is essential during pregnancy for the health of mother and baby, and the process of bringing a new life into the world can introduce issues that are well-beyond the scope of this book. So first and foremost, consult with your healthcare team about the best course of action for you when you're pregnant.

Chapter Fourteen

Raw Food Claims, Myths, Promises and Fantasies

If you're researching raw foods at all, sooner or later you'll run into people making some pretty interesting claims and promises. More than a few warnings get passed around as well. The following describes my personal experiences with these claims.

The Fears

Rotting Teeth

No, my teeth aren't rotting. In fact, this warning just seems like far-fetched fear-mongering to me. I recently visited the dentist after a two-year hiatus and what did she say?

"Your teeth are in perfect condition."

Here's the deal: As everyone knows, if you eat a lot of sweets and don't care for your teeth properly, you'll probably have issues with cavities or worse. If you maintain dental hygiene and eat a varied, balanced, healthy diet, I don't see why eating raw vegan would increase the rate of tooth decay. It seems to me that cutting out all those processed sugars would actually *decrease* decay. Unless you fall into the trap of eating a lot of dried fruit, I don't see anything to worry about here. I'm not a dentist, but let's just apply a little common sense. Avoid excess sugar, take care of your teeth (floss, floss, floss)—and don't forget to check in with the dentist regularly. Tongue scraping and neem oil are terrific for oral health.

Wasting Away

Maybe you've come across photos of raw vegan, skeletal-type folks who look like they're on their last legs. Yes, these people exist, and possibly people with eating disorders are drawn to the raw food diet (along with other diets). I can't really say.

As with any diet, if you don't eat enough food, you'll lose weight—and possibly, *too* much weight. This is one reason I scowl just a little when I hear raw food enthusiasts promise that you can eat a raw vegan diet with only a knife and a cutting board. It's my belief that folks who experience excessive weight loss when they switch to eating raw are probably just taking in fewer calories than they were before and aren't taking advantage of the amazing variety of nutritious raw foods available.

While, generally speaking, whole foods are less calorie-dense than processed items, some ingredients in typical raw food diets are not low in calories at all, such as nuts, seeds and oils.

When I first went raw I was afraid of losing weight, as I had a tendency to be very thin. As my body became cleaner, it began to be very clear on what it needed to stay healthy. I actually *gained* a little weight going from the Standard American Diet to raw foods, and now I've remained at a very healthy weight without issue or monitoring for many years.

Hair Falling Out

This was another really scary myth for me! Several years prior to going raw, out of acne desperation, I finally agreed to go on Accutane. THAT made my hair fall out! I was on the drug for only five weeks, watching my dermatologist throw up his hands and shrug about whether or not my thinning mane would ever return. I stopped taking it and my hair eventually grew back, although it took years. Naturally, when I heard the warning that my hair might thin out on a raw food diet, I was terrified.

This myth is obviously related to the fear that you're not going to get enough nutrients to grow strong nails and maintain a head of hair. If you think about it, though, this makes no sense at all. How are you going to up your intake of uncooked (read: alive and unaltered) whole foods and get *fewer* nutrients than you did eating pizza, hamburgers and french fries? As noted, cooking generally destroys about half of the protein in foods, and many other nutrients as well.

No, my hair did not fall out eating raw food. If anything, it got thicker.

The Promises

Perfect Skin

To be entirely honest, this is one of the main reasons I went raw: perfect (or at least drastically improved) skin. Having dealt with pretty severe acne issues for most of my adult life, the skin thing was really, *really* motivating for me.

My skin *has* improved by leaps and bounds. I had so many people tell me, "Oh, your skin will be perfectly clear when you eat this way!"

Well, okay, no. And believe me, when it comes to clear skin, if you've heard of it, I've tried it! I've attempted everything from completely removing the oil from my diet (I've never felt worse and my skin was *terrible*) to taking Accutane, birth control pills and other pharmaceuticals and everything in between. Most of the time my skin is clear of blemishes now, although I do still experience hormonal breakouts periodically. Lately this is quite rare for me. I believe getting enough good-quality sleep has drastically improved the quality of my skin.

And what about wrinkles? Yes, I am still getting some of these. At fifty years old, I've got a few fine lines around my eyes. That's really about it, though. I do not yet have the forehead wrinkles, lip creases or "marionette lines" I see on some women's faces my age. Just to be clear, though, I have also been quite the sun-phobe for most of my life and am adamant about sunscreen, hats, umbrellas and generally staying out of the direct sun as much as possible (which many people will tell you is unhealthy; I do try to strike some kind of a balance here).

I have no question that the raw vegan diet plays a role in healthier skin, but so will other factors such as exercise, sleep, stress and your own genetic predispositions.

No Gray Hair

Here's one I was pretty excited about: I'd read about retaining natural hair color and also about gray hair *returning* to its natural color. It's pretty hard to tell what would have happened if I hadn't started eating raw vegan, but I can tell you that while I still do have some gray hairs, they don't seem to be multiplying very quickly.

When melatonin production ceases in cells in the hair follicles, hair appears gray. Many of the factors that impact production of melatonin are nutritionally related, so it makes sense that we're in great shape as raw vegans for retaining our natural hair color.

Additional factors that can influence melatonin production are B12 deficiency, thyroid imbalance, stress, toxic buildup in the body and hormonal imbalances. If we are watching our B12 and eating a varied, raw organic diet, we are automatically cleansing and supporting continual healing and balance in all body systems. One result of a healthy body is shiny, healthy hair!

Perfect Eyesight

One of the exciting promises I heard was that people's vision improved and they didn't need their glasses anymore. You will probably also read something about improved eyesight on a raw vegan diet.[80] This may have to do with increased nutrient absorption or the cumulative effects of a generally healthy lifestyle. In the latter case you can't go wrong, even if it doesn't improve your eyesight.

Here's my experience: I already had great vision, so I assumed eating raw would ensure this for years to come. You should have heard me brag about my better-than-20/20 vision for years and years! When I went to see my eye doctor in my late thirties and he told me that at age forty my vision would start to deteriorate, I laughed all the way out of the office. Not me!

Well . . . As soon as I turned forty-three, menus started to blur and I could no longer make out the streets on my map of L.A. I finally swallowed my pride and broke down and bought reading glasses. I pull them out to read any super-fine print.

It's virtually impossible to tell whether or not my vision would be worse (or the same) eating differently. Who knows? I also typically spend several hours a day on the computer and reading books, which is clearly a strain on my eyes. Both my parents wore glasses to read and most of my peers are experiencing this "hold-the-phone-at-arm's-length" phenomenon just like I am, no matter what they eat.

Increased Energy

Yes, hands down, this is true. I have tons of energy, even if I don't sleep enough. I used to wind down about four o'clock in the afternoon and then get that no-sleep headache even after only one night of not enough sleep.

No more. Unless I'm under the weather, I've got massive amounts of energy and will do cartwheels across the room (literally—if it's big enough). I just can't stop myself! Although I'm usually not a runner, many times at the gym I'll run for a while just to release some of that extra oomph.

Increased energy: yes.

Moles and Scars Disappearing

Here's one promise I've seen no evidence of whatsoever.

While my skin tends to heal quickly if I have a wound and I never really scarred all that badly, this appears to be no different than before I started eating raw food. None of my old skin imperfections have disappeared or faded, either. Dang.

Never Get Sick Again!

As I described previously, I have a long history of being sick. A lot. Most of my childhood was spent in the hospital. Because of my atypical health history, it's really hard to judge this raw food promise based on my experience. But what I can say is that I'm worlds away from where I was in my pre-raw days, when I'd get sick all the time and take weeks to fully recover.

Yes, I still periodically catch colds, and sometimes I'll have a cough hang around for a while post-infection. The difference is that now I don't get as sick as I used to, I heal much more quickly and I do not contract as many illnesses as I did before, even though I work with babies and small children, who seem to always be drooling or sneezing on me.

I've discovered that supporting my immune system is key. Probiotics are critical and if I skimp on sleep over a period of a few days, I seem to become more vulnerable to catching something. But for me, this has always been true, raw or not.

Now I'm ultra-tuned-in to my body and can tell quite quickly when my immune system is running low and I'm fighting something. Most of the time I can nip a cold in the bud by laying low for a couple of days and juicing, drinking herbal mixtures and generally resting up. But if I make the opposite choice and head to the gym (I can be very stubborn!) or stay out late one more night, I'm often heading right into Cold City.

Decreased Inflammation

Here's some great news! My chiropractor will attest to the fact that because I eat raw, plant-based foods, I do not encounter typical issues related to inflammation. Hence, my herniated discs give me little to no trouble at all, although I definitely do have periods of aches and pains when I don't treat my back kindly.

After looking at my MRI results, I had two chiropractors and a physical therapist ask me how I was even walking around "in my condition." The answer is simple: my back is no longer inflamed. Avoiding inflammation is also great for warding off a host of other issues. Chronic low-grade systemic inflammation plays a critical role in many diseases. Arthritis, lupus, asthma (also key for me), Crohn's disease, diabetes, gum disease, heart disease, pulmonary fibrosis and cancer are a few, but there are many more. Inflammation is a killer. My chiropractor has informed me that if it weren't for my diet, I'd be in his office daily asking for relief.

♥   ♥   ♥

I've touched on a variety of fears and potential benefits of a raw vegan diet in this chapter, and for the most part I've tried to stick to my own experiences. The truth is that everyone is unique and there are countless factors that affect how our bodies respond to any change, including to the introduction of raw food. No matter what anyone says—including me—your job is to pay attention to what's happening to your own body on (or off) the raw vegan diet. This means periodically checking in with your physician to ensure that your nutrient levels are where they need to be. But it also means listening to and observing your own body. Your body will give you strong clues as to what's working and what's not. Experimenting with the benefits of raw food can be a great way to train yourself to listen to what your body is telling you. We receive far more feedback from our inner voice than we realize. Reconnecting with that wisdom is one of the greatest gifts we can give ourselves.

Chapter Fifteen

How to Stay Raw
Without Going Nuts

I had a lot of reasons to go raw vegan. I loved animals. I had grave concerns about the environment. I experienced a lot of physical pain and discomfort and craved excellent health. And I enjoyed internal calm and mental acuity. Eating raw was an excellent fit for me in all areas.

But one of the primary reasons I *stayed* raw, day after day, year after year, and was able to say no to cheese puffs, donuts, bread, cheese and cheesecake (which I liked as much as the next person) was because when I ate raw, I felt so good that no cooked lemon bar was worth the brain fog, rash, stomachache, pimple or food coma that inevitably followed.

Maybe I was blessed in a way. My gluten, processed sugar and lactose intolerances, herniated discs and hormonal imbalances actually caused me physical discomfort and had disturbing effects on my appearance when I consumed the wrong foods. My body's alarm system made it very easy to want to avoid that pain, and when I ignored it, I often got hit right where it hurt me most: my vanity.

Choices

When I first went raw I wasn't aware of all the menu options out there. You may find, as I did, that in the beginning everything around you seems to be cooked or non-vegan. You may initially feel hemmed in by an apparent lack of choices. For my own part, before I'd established some go-to standards to rely on, it was admittedly a bit tough. Make it easy on yourself and always have a stash of raw vegan snacks or easy meals stashed away. Even just a cereal mix or almond butter/raw crackers cache can keep you from ordering a pizza on those evenings when you come home late with a growling stomach.

There's a false perception that eating raw is a very restrictive way of eating, using very limited ingredients. I fell prey to that belief myself when I started out.

What I soon realized, though, is that while, yes, you're eliminating *some* foods (and a bunch of food-like products), most people's regular menus are made up of only about ten items anyway. Think about what you usually eat on a daily basis. What are some of the typical foods on the Standard American Diet? Chicken, beef, fish, rice, bread and maybe a wimpy salad once in a while—rinse and repeat.

If you're exploring raw foods and eating seasonal offerings, you're actually exponentially *expanding* your ingredient choices rather than limiting them. Although it may not feel that way at first. For my own part, I even ate some cooked food here and there in the beginning, when I felt stuck without something raw on hand. The thing is, I couldn't help but notice that as time went by and I ate progressively "cleaner," when I *did* eat something cooked I felt even worse than I used to.

This encouraged me to continue seeking out new raw vegan options. Eventually I found I could eat a wonderfully diverse, healthy diet rich in nutrients, without expending immense effort. I noticed I began to choose raw over cooked food simply because I loved it and I loved the way I felt when eating it.

This, too, is how I hope it will be for you. One of the goals of this book has been to make the process easier, and to show you that you don't have to go it alone. With that in mind, let's look at a few other ways to keep yourself on the straight and narrow as you follow the raw vegan path to health.

Side-Stepping Temptation

For me, sticking with raw food is also about not putting myself in temptation's path. If I see an ice cream sandwich or a slice of cheesecake, I'll want to eat it. I *won't* eat it, but I'll want to.

At the beginning of my journey with raw food, I *would* eat it, until I got tired of the diarrhea, rashes, brain fog and food comas. Knowing that I can get raw cheesecake and ice cream that far exceeds conventional types is terrific, but if there's a Twinkie sitting in front of me, heck yeah, I still want it!

In order to avoid negative repercussions in both the long and short term, we pass up lots of things. Saying no to unhealthy treats is no different. I don't buy every cute pair of shoes I spot or lunge out into traffic when I want to cross the street, just like I don't eat everything that looks good.

Passing on our old favorites, however, can be the toughest change. For me, the raw version of mac and cheese is great, but I'll never forget the amazing day-glow orange, plastic yumminess of those Kraft noodles in the blue box. So generally, though it doesn't have a huge effect on me anymore, I just try not to be around it—temptation can be powerful!

Something I find helpful is to slowly collect a few new favorites to replace old cravings. If I've got a rare craving for sweets, I whip up some cookies or banana ice cream, or eat a date. If I'm in dire want of bread, I've got my great raisin bread I can put together in ten minutes (plus dehydrator time).

Sure, the substitutes might not be exactly the same as your old go-to's, but they certainly can hit the spot. And if you want to get really fancy, you can probably find a recipe that will get close to your old faves. Pretty soon the substitutes become the real thing, and you crave those instead; it's truly all in what we're used to. I can honestly say that when I look at a dessert tray or bakery case, most of the time these items don't even register in my brain as food anymore—no kidding!

Staying Inspired and Motivated

When times get tough, the tough get motivated! Bookmark this page so that when it seems just too annoying, difficult, boring or dumb to keep going, you'll have some much-needed support at the ready. Here are some of the tricks and tips I've used when I needed that extra push to stay motivated. I'm sure you'll dream up your own to add to this list as you progress on your raw journey!

Recipes Old and New

Create a favorite recipe binder and add to your collection as you go. I've kept a couple of these for years and go back again and again to these favorite recipes. Sometimes I paste in recipes I've cut from magazines or print them off the Internet and put them in plastic sleeves, adding them to my binder collection.

Go spelunking for some tantalizing new recipes. I highly recommend finding raw vegan recipe websites with amazing photographs. These really get me chomping at the bit to get back into the kitchen. Rawmazing.com, as mentioned previously, is one of my favorites.

While buying a lot of recipe books is not what gets me going, I do like having a few great ones for simple recipes. My current faves are Alissa Cohen's *Living on Live Food,* Cara Brotman and Markus Rothkranz's *Love on a Plate,* Laurel Anderson's *Wild Plate,* and one for fancier desserts: Café Gratitude's *Sweet Gratitude: A New World of Raw Desserts.*

Premade Raw Foods

Buy some premade raw foods and try recreating them yourself. This allows you to enjoy a premade treat (quite a relief sometimes—though usually not as healthy as ones you'll prepare yourself), while providing you with new recipe ideas. While the proportions are not listed on the ingredients lists, raw food is very forgiving. Sometimes my version comes out better than the packaged original!

Social Media

Join a Facebook or other social media group for raw food. There's never any shortage of discussions going on, and recipe sharing abounds. You can also start your own Facebook group. This takes about four minutes to set up and gives you the advantage of being able to invite any of your friends who may be interested in raw food.

There's also the option of joining or starting a Meetup group. I've done both, and Meetups can be a whole lot of fun. Though I'd warn participants away from engaging with the ranting, judgmental arguments that sometimes erupt over the minutiae of the raw food lifestyle, having a community of folks who understand what you're doing can be very supportive.

Get Friends Involved

Call a friend. Do you have a good friend or family member who could be your food lifeline? The two of you could spend a few minutes brainstorming menu ideas. Sometimes two is more fun than one, even if your friend isn't raw vegan; just having a supportive person who loves you is all it takes.

You could also invite some friends over for a meal or snacks. (This works for getting your house clean too!) I find that even when I'm bored of prepping food for myself, I often enjoy making food for others.

Restaurants

Enjoy a delicious meal at a raw restaurant, if that's an option. Again, this will give you a break from food prep, and you might come away inspired. I call it a "reset" and consider it part of my raw food journey. Ask if the restaurant has a paper menu you can keep, and see if there's anything on it you'd like to whip up at home. You can keep a binder of take-out menus as well, for extra inspiration when you need it.

Steal from the Pros

Watch a cooking show, or maybe even one of my own favorites, *Kitchen Nightmares*. Even though these shows are about *cooking*, they often inspire me to get into the kitchen and whip something up. Sometimes I'll narrate as I make the dish as if I was on the show myself. Why not?

Consider also browsing a magazine for cooked recipes that you can try "raw-veganizing." I enjoy this challenge every once in a while and have come up with some fun new raw renditions.

Raw Chefs

Take advantage of all the free education out there in the form of YouTube videos uploaded by raw chefs. Ani Phyo, who I had the honor of meeting, is one of my favorites. You can also check out Juliano Brotman, Markus Rothkranz, David Wolfe, Matt Monarch, Angela Stokes, FullyRaw Kristina, Jenny Ross, Laura Miller and Philip and Casey McCluskey. Any one of them (or someone else) might float your boat and spark an interest with their videos. Just do a search for "raw vegan" and see what comes up!

This may even inspire you to start creating your own videos and posting them on YouTube. It's kind of like cooking for company, but the company just doesn't happen to be sitting on your couch.

Mix It Up

To use a cliché that's actually so true: variety is the spice of life. There are many ideas you can come up with to invite spontaneity and serendipity into your raw regimen. For example, pick one food category a week and try a new recipe. Sometimes just this can pull you out of a rut.

Order a CSA box. This is one of my favorite things! Sometimes I just eat the food straight out of the box, and other times it will inspire me to do an Internet search for recipes featuring the ingredients in that week's box.

Take a trip to a store you've never been to and see if you can find a few items that look enticing. An unfamiliar seasonal fruit or veggie might catch your eye. I remember when I moved to L.A. and spotted dragon fruit for the first time. I literally did a little dance of delight in the middle of Whole Foods and called a stranger over to take a look; I'd never seen anything so beautiful!

Take a Break

Take some time to reflect on what might be feeling overwhelming or stressful in your life in general.

Instead of serving as a relaxing wind-down, preparing food— raw or not—can sometimes feel like the last straw on top of a too-busy day. We all experience periods of increased activity and the desire for social engagement followed by more fallow periods when we find ourselves craving rest and rejuvenation. Food may simply be the scapegoat for other frustrations. Sometimes we may find that our exasperation has less to do with our diet and more to do with larger life patterns. Creating some time and space for self-connection and care, such as a free afternoon, an hour of yoga or a guided meditation, can shift everything.

In any case, when it comes to food frustration, the bigger picture is often worth exploring.

Maybe, however, for whatever reason, you just need a few days off without thinking about food, period. This might be a great time to indulge in various delicious juices and smoothies for a day or two without pressuring yourself to create any "dishes." Not only will you survive a couple of liquid-only days, you'll be giving your body an additional cleansing boost as well.

Whenever I run out of food and don't feel like going to the store, I'll call it a "smoothie fast" and get on with whatever I'm doing. I always notice my skin becoming extra soft and clear during these times. Eventually I tire of liquids, however, and get hungry for something else—and hunger is a great motivator to get to the store and back into the kitchen!

Food Overwhelm & Choice

As with any other commitment fatigue, such as that New Year's commitment to go to the gym on a regular basis, there may be times when you simply don't want to eat raw vegan. You may feel trapped and just plain angry about it. Truly, eating raw vegan *can* seem annoying at times.

Remember, though, that moods come and go, and you'll weather this one, too. Particularly if other things in your life feel stressful, preparing a raw vegan meal might feel overwhelming and just too difficult. When you're hungry, in a hurry or away from home, trying to find something edible can be irritating. Sometimes you just want to drive to the closest grocery store or fast-food joint like everybody else and pick up some taquitos. It's not only that you'd rather not whip up some raw tortillas, it's that you're mad about *having* to.

What to do?

First of all, simply allow the mood. It's going to be there whether you resist it or not, so save yourself some time and energy and accept it instead of resisting. Let it pass through, just watching it rather than adding content like, "Yeah I knew this was a bad idea!

It's too hard!" Your mood will be gone soon enough, and then you'll remember why you love eating this way.

In the meantime, exercise patience with yourself. Give the feeling of food overwhelm some space. It deserves love too!

It can be helpful to remember that ultimately the way you eat is up to you. You *can* pull up to McDonald's and order a burger and fries if you really want to. No one's stopping you but yourself. (In fact, it might even *help* if it serves as a reminder for how your body responds to that kind of meal.)

Just remembering that this is a *choice* can be helpful, and that you're committed to this for a reason.

Try reminding yourself of the following during times of duress:

- How great you feel eating this way

- How crappy you felt *not* eating this way

- How good you *look* eating raw

- How cooked food sticks to your teeth (I HATE that!)

- . . . and whatever else you find that you love about eating raw vegan food.

Remember that you're the one in control—not the food.

When feeling overwhelmed with *anything*, much less your dietary choices, you've got a perfect opportunity to take a step back, give yourself a breather and check in with your intuitive wisdom. Most of us will find any reason we can to be hard on ourselves. So cutting ourselves some slack in moments like these can actually give us just the clarity we need to see the way forward.

Conclusion

What we eat is a powerful force in our lives. Choosing what to eat becomes an empowering honor when we realize that it is in our realm of control to select foods that create a force for disconnection, disease and ill-health or one of optimal healing, clarity, awareness and transformation.

The label "Living Foods" is not a marketing term. It's literally the truth. While an animal's life force leaves immediately upon being killed and its flesh begins to decompose soon after, a plant, when harvested, continues to live for a period of time afterwards. When we eat the plant, we are eating a live organism, and we absorb its life force into our own. When we consume dead and rotting foods, we absorb that dead energy and zap our body's vitality. Living foods *add* to our vitality.

Given the right conditions, as the living seed can be planted and grow into the healthiest, mature version of itself, so do we mature into the highest versions of ourselves if we are supplied the right conditions. Many people find that raw food is indeed one of these "right conditions."

Unlike traditional "diets," diet pills or formulas that rely on unsustainable self-deprivation, providing the body with the right conditions for recovery and rejuvenation creates a stable foundation for all kinds of true healing to happen naturally. No calorie-counting, no pills and no programs, just real food and real healing.

The decision to cease inputting unnatural, lifeless foods into our systems and to replace them with healthy living foods can be a massive step towards reconnection with our bodies and our true selves. By giving our systems the right conditions for healing, they can begin to clear out all of the junk—and that's when we start experiencing what it feels like to be alive and well in our bodies.

Suddenly those little discomforts register and we can act on them. We notice when we're hungry and when we're full, when this or that food isn't what our body wants. We discover that our system is really craving true health, and that to eat *well* is a gift we give ourselves: an act of love.

And then something magical happens. We begin to notice that under all of the static and thought, from a place of deep wisdom, our hearts are speaking to us. As we act on what we hear, we begin— perhaps for the first time in our lives—to trust our bodies and our intuition.

We experience our inherent truth.

We reconnect.

Eating food is a reflection of and a metaphor for what we are consuming in all areas of our lives. As we start to make that connection, perhaps then we also re-evaluate our personal care products, our cleaning products, our recycling habits and what we allow into our space and consciousness in terms of clutter on all levels—including news, social media, and other people's energy. *We start to value ourselves.* We notice that we no longer align with destructive energies and they fall away on their own. We start to see where things are out of integrity for us and do a complete declutter in our lives, in the words of Marie Kondo, keeping only "what sparks joy." We begin to experience connection not only to our bodies and ourselves, but to others, to our community, to the planet, and to our role in universal wellness. We become stewards and emissaries of Health, Truth and Love.

The transformative effects begin to multiply exponentially.

Suddenly, we notice our perception is different. We're more clear, our bodies begin to lose the pounds we couldn't seem to shed (or gain the ones we couldn't keep on) and our entire beings and lives start to take on their natural shapes, externally and internally.

The course of our lives shifts as we begin to remember who we are and what we're here for on every plane: Love!

Reconnection. Rejuvenation. Transformation.

Food is our connection to our mother—the Earth. Without her, there is no life. As we are nourished by our mothers *in utero*, after birth we continue to be nourished by mother Earth. But with our birth into the world there eventually comes a choice: which sustenance will we choose? That which fosters disconnection, malnourishment and disease? Or true nourishment close to the source—that which will truly nurture us and connect us with our roots, our intuition and our wisdom?

It's up to us.

With raw food, you're embarking on a road less-traveled, and with some perseverance, you may well find it to be one of the most rewarding of your life. You're moving towards health, joy, connection with the Earth, and Oneness. What could be more worthwhile?

Eat up, friends, and enjoy! May you partake of life in the deepest way. In love, friendship, vitality, alignment, connection, clarity and transformation: I wish you well!

The word "raw" is, of course, "war" spelled backwards. The power of raw food is that it is actually nothing less than an appetizingly concealed weapon. With every trip to the market, every dish we create and every mouth we serve, we wield the power to march forward in a peaceful coalition of kindness. But make no mistake: what we are engaged in is a vital war for our very lives against forces threatening not only our personal health and consciousness, but the planet and the fate of all life. Whether we realize it or not, when we *don't* make conscious food choices, we are lobbing a grenade for disease, over-use of pharmaceuticals, consumerism, animal cruelty, farming with poisons, pollution, habitat destruction, and climate change. Conversely, each bite of living foods is a peaceful march towards health, sustainability, independence, interdependence, animal welfare, habitat preservation, organic farming, planetary health and LOVE.

Let's turn not just the word around, but ourselves, the world, and the course of history as well. Let's create something beautiful for all beings from kindness, peace and Love. Now is the time!

Recipes

W orld-renowned raw chef, Ron Russell, of the award-wining SunCafe Organic in Los Angeles has graciously shared with us some spectacular recipes to get started. Enjoy!

♥   ♥   ♥

WALDORF SALAD (serves 4)

3 cups	Apples, large (medium chopped)
1 cup	Celery (small chopped)
½ cup	Raisins
1 teaspoon	Cinnamon
1 tablespoon	Pecans or walnuts (diced)
3 tablespoons	Sunflower mayo (see recipe below)

Toss salad ingredients with mayo in a bowl. Top with cinnamon stick for decoration.

♥   ♥   ♥

Recipes courtesy of Chef Ron Russell of SunCafe Organic.

CHARD AND SPINACH SALAD w/GODDESS DRESSING
(serves 4–6)

4 cups	Chard (ribs stripped out, packed)
2 cups	Spinach (packed)
½ cup	Cherry tomatoes or chopped tomatoes

Chop chard and spinach into thin strips. Add desired amount of dressing (see recipe below) and top with tomatoes.

♥   ♥   ♥

SUNFLOWER MAYO

1 cup	Sunflower seeds (soaked and drained)
1 tablespoon	Olive oil
3 tablespoons	Lemon juice
1 cup	Water
1 tablespoon	Apple cider vinegar
1 teaspoon	Salt
1	Clove garlic

Mix all ingredients in blender until smooth.

♥   ♥   ♥

KALE AND SPINACH DIP

2 cups	Spinach (packed)
2 cups	Kale (ribs stripped out)
1 tablespoon	Lemon juice
¼ cup	Onion
1 tablespoon	Nutritional yeast
1 tablespoon	Dill (fresh)

Recipes courtesy of Chef Ron Russell of SunCafe Organic.

½ teaspoon	Sea salt
1	Avocado (peeled and pitted)
1 Pinch	Cayenne pepper

Mix in food processor until smooth. Serve with fresh vegetables, raw crackers or on small cabbage leaves.

♥　　♥　　♥

GODDESS DRESSING

½ cup	Raw sesame seeds
¾ cup	Water
2 tablespoons	Bragg apple cider vinegar
2 tablespoons	Lemon juice
1 teaspoon	Coconut aminos
1 tablespoon	Fresh dill
1	Garlic clove, small
1	Date or 1 tablespoon coconut nectar
Sea salt to taste	

Blend all ingredients except dill until completely smooth. Add dill and pulse blender 2x.

♥　　♥　　♥

SUNFLOWER SCRAMBLE (serves 2–4)

1½ cups	Sunflower seeds (soaked and drained)
1 cup	Zucchini (rough chopped)
¾ teaspoon	Turmeric
1 teaspoon	Cumin
2 tablespoons	Cilantro, chopped
2 teaspoons	Nutritional yeast
¾ teaspoon	Sea salt
Dash of pepper	

Recipes courtesy of Chef Ron Russell of SunCafe Organic.

1 tablespoon   Water

Mix everything in a food processor. Add additional water until desired "scrambled" texture achieved (do not blend into a paste). Transfer mixture into a bowl and then add the following ingredients.

4	Sun-dried tomatoes (finely diced)
½ cup	Tomatoes (diced)
½ cup	Red pepper (diced)
½ cup	Celery (fine chopped)
1	Green onion (chopped)

Combine vegetables with scramble and mix with a spoon. Serve.

♥   ♥   ♥

TOMATO BASIL SOUP (serves 1–2)

4 cups	Tomatoes
½ cup	Sun-dried tomatoes (hydrated)
1	Celery stalk
1	Carrot (small)
½ cup	Basil leaves (fresh)
1	Garlic clove
½ teaspoon	Sea salt
½ teaspoon	Pepper
¾ cup	Water

Rough chop ingredients and blend until smooth. Option: add more fresh basil and diced avocado for garnish.

♥   ♥   ♥

ZUCCHINI OCEAN TACOS (serves 4)

1	Zucchini (medium)
1 tablespoon	Dulse or nori (minced)

Recipes courtesy of Chef Ron Russell of SunCafe Organic.

½ teaspoon	Cumin
½	Garlic clove (minced)
¼ teaspoon	Chili powder
¼ teaspoon	Sea salt
Pinch of pepper	

Cut zucchini lengthwise into eighths. Place zucchini in a sealable container and add spices. Marinate for 2 hours.

Assemble

½ cup	Cabbage (chopped)
4	Romaine lettuce leaves
4	Cilantro sprigs
¼ cup	Salsa
Option: Guacamole	

Fill Romaine lettuce leave "taco shells" with zucchini, cabbage, salsa, and one cilantro sprig per taco. Top with spicy lime cream (recipe follows).

♥　　♥　　♥

SPICY LIME CREAM

1 cup	Sunflower seeds (soaked)
¼ cup	Lime juice
1 tablespoon	Apple cider vinegar
½ teaspoon	Cayenne
½ teaspoon	Sea salt
¾ cup	Water (as needed)

Blend all ingredients in blender or food processor until smooth.

♥　　♥　　♥

Recipes courtesy of Chef Ron Russell of SunCafe Organic.

BASIC SALSA

¼ cup	Tomatoes (diced)
1 teaspoon	Lemon juice
2 tablespoons	Onion (diced)
Sea salt to taste	
Pinch of cayenne pepper	

Combine and mix ingredients.

♥　　♥　　♥

BURGER *(serves 4)*

2 cups	Sunflower seeds, soaked and drained
½ cup	Sun-dried tomatoes, soaked and drained
2	Romaine leaves
1 cup	Carrots (grated/juice pressed out or pulp)
2 tablespoons	Onions
2 teaspoons	Cumin
½ teaspoon	Coriander
1½ teaspoons	Onion powder
1 tablespoon	Nutritional yeast
1 teaspoon	Turmeric
¾ teaspoon	Sea salt
Option: Dehydrate 6–8 hours	

Put all ingredients except romaine leaves into food processor. Run until sunflower seeds become crumbly. Form into small patties. Serve room temperature or dehydrate to warm. Assemble patties sandwiched between two romaine leaves. Options: serve with mayo, thin onion slice, raw pickles.

♥　　♥　　♥

Recipes courtesy of Chef Ron Russell of SunCafe Organic.

MISO SOUP (serves 1–2)

1½ tablespoon	Red or brown miso paste
1 teaspoon	Onion powder
1 tablespoon	Green onion
½ cup	Bok choy, chard, or collard greens (chopped into small, thin strips)
2 cups	Water

¼ Nori sheet cut into 1-inch squares OR ¼ teaspoon wakame

In high-powered blender, blend miso, onion powder, and water until warm. Add nori and other vegetables and serve.

♥   ♥   ♥

LEMON BARS (serves 4)

1 cup	Soft dates (pitted)
¾ cup	Raw shredded coconut
¾ cup	Shredded carrots
½ cup	Raisins
¼ cup	Lemon juice
1 tablespoon	Lemon zest
Pinch sea salt	

Mix all ingredients well in a bowl. Form into bars or balls. Refrigerate 1 hour. Option: roll balls in shredded coconut.

♥   ♥   ♥

SIMPLE STRAWBERRY SHORTCAKE (serves 2)

Recipes courtesy of Chef Ron Russell of SunCafe Organic.

2	Ripe bananas
1 cup	Raw shredded coconut
1 cup	Strawberries

With a fork, mash bananas with coconut. Form into mini cake. Mash strawberries and use to top banana cake. Option: add 1 teaspoon of coconut nectar or date syrup to strawberries to sweeten.

♥   ♥   ♥

Recipes courtesy of Chef Ron Russell of SunCafe Organic.

Resources

General Books

Balch, Phyllis A. *Prescription for Nutritional Healing: the A-to-Z Guide to Supplements*. New York, NY: Penguin Group, 2010.

Boutenko, Victoria. *Green for Life: the Updated Classic on Green Smoothie Nutrition*. Berkeley, CA: North Atlantic, 2010.

Campbell, T. Colin, and Thomas M. Campbell. *The China Study: the Most Comprehensive Study of Nutrition Ever Conducted and the Startling Implications for Diet, Weight Loss and Long-Term Health*. Dallas, TX: BenBella Books, Inc., 2017.

Campbell, T. Colin, and Howard Jacobson. *Whole: Rethinking the Science of Nutrition*. Dallas, TX: BenBella Books, 2014.

Cohen, Alissa. *Living on Live Food*. Kittery, Me.: Cohen Pub. Co., 2009.

Eisenstein, Charles. *The Yoga of Eating: Transcending Diets and Dogma to Nourish the Natural Self*. Washington, D.C.: NewTrends Publishington, 2003.

Fife, Bruce. *The Coconut Oil Miracle*. 5th ed. New York: Avery, 2014.

Fitzgerald, Randall. *The Hundred-Year Lie: How to Protect Yourself from the Chemicals That Are Destroying Your Health*. New York: Plume, 2007.

Gagné, Steve. *Food Energetics: The Spiritual, Emotional, and Nutritional Power of What We Eat*. Rochester, VT: Healing Arts Press, 2008.

Greger, Michael, and Gene Stone. *How Not to Die: Discover the Foods Scientifically Proven to Prevent and Reverse Disease*. New York: Flatiron, 2015.

Harden, Christy. *Guided by Your Own Stars: Connect with the Inner Voice and Discover Your Dreams*. Anna Maria, FL: Maurice Bassett, 2014.

Hawthorne, Mark. *Striking at the Roots: a Practical Guide to Animal Activism - 10th Anniversary Edition - New ... Tactics, New Technology*. Hampshire, UK: Changemakers Books, 2018.

Newkirk, Ingrid. *Making Kind Choices: Everyday Ways to Enhance Your Life through Earth-and Animal-Friendly Living*. New York, NY: St. Martins Griffin, 2005.

Shiva, Vandana. *Soil, Not Oil: Climate Change, Peak Oil and Food Insecurity*. London: Zed Books, 2016.

Siegel-Maier, Karyn. *The Naturally Clean Home*. North Adams, MA: Storey, 2009.

Sunstein, Cass, and Martha Nussbaum, eds. *Animal Rights: Current Debates and New Directions*. New York, NY: Oxford University Press, 2004.

Cookbooks

Adrian, Ann, and Judith Dennis. *Herbal Tea Book*. San Francisco, CA: Health Pub. Co., 1976.

Anderson, Laurel. *Wild Plate: Modern Living Cuisine*. Olympia, WA: Laurel Anderson, 2013.

Boutenko, Sergei, and Valya Boutenko. *Fresh: the Ultimate Live-Food Cookbook*. Berkeley, CA: North Atlantic Books, 2008.

Brotman, Cara, and Markus Rothkranz. *Love on a Plate: the Gourmet Uncookbook: Raw Vegan Versions of the Most Favorite Meals in the World*. United States: Rothkranz Publishing, 2014.

Drakes Press. *Fermentation for Beginners: the Step-by-Step Guide to Fermentation and Probiotic Foods*. Berkeley, CA: Drakes Press, 2013.

Cornbleet, Jennifer. *Raw Food Made Easy for 1 or 2 People*. Summertown, TN: Book Publishing, 2012.

Johnson, Mark, and Kim Johnson. *Rapid Raw Revised: Fast Raw Food Recipes*. True Living Health Products, 2014.

Kenney, Matthew, Sarma Melngailis, and Jen Karetnick. *Raw Food, Real World: 100 Recipes to Get the Glow*. New York, NY: William Morrow, 2011.

Wolfe, David. *Eating for Beauty*. Berkeley, CA: North Atlantic Books, 2009.

Films

Fat, Sick & Nearly Dead, 2010.
Forks Over Knives, 2011.
Simply Raw, 2009.

Notes

Preface

[1] Fife, Bruce. *The Coconut Oil Miracle*. 5th ed. New York: Avery, 2014.
[2] Boutenko, Victoria. *Green for Life: The Updated Classic on Green Smoothie Nutrition*. Berkeley, CA: North Atlantic, 2010.

Chapter One: The Raw Food Manifesto

[3] Gagné, Steve. *Food Energetics: The Spiritual, Emotional, and Nutritional Power of What We Eat*. Rochester, VT: Healing Arts Press, 2008.
[4] "Stephanie Seneff, Ph.D - High Intensity Health: Mike Mutzel." High Intensity Health | Mike Mutzel. Accessed March 12, 2020. https://highintensityhealth.com/stephanie-seneff-Ph.D./.
[5] Gagné, Steve. *Food Energetics: The Spiritual, Emotional, and Nutritional Power of What We Eat*. Rochester, VT: Healing Arts Press, 2008.

Chapter Two: A Deeper Look Into Food Decisions

[6] Medscape Log In. Accessed February 26, 2020. http://www.medscape.com/medline/abstract/21135297.
[7] "Adult Obesity Facts." Centers for Disease Control and Prevention. Centers for Disease Control and Prevention, February 27, 2020. https://www.cdc.gov/obesity/data/adult.html

[8] Campbell, T. Colin, and Howard Jacobson. *Whole: Rethinking the Science of Nutrition*. Dallas, TX: BenBella Books, 2014.

[9] "2015-2020 Dietary Guidelines." Home of the Office of Disease Prevention and Health Promotion. Accessed March 15, 2020. https://health.gov/our-work/food-nutrition/2015-2020-dietary-guidelines These guidelines are informed by the USDA's *Scientific Report of the 2015 Dietary Guidelines Advisory Committee*, available here: http://health.gov/dietaryguidelines/2015-scientific-report/pdfs/scientific-report-of-the-2015-dietary-guidelines-advisory-committee.pdf

[10] To readers interested in exploring the food science behind recommendations for a plant-based diet and its healing properties, I highly recommend the following book: Greger, Michael, and Gene Stone. *How Not to Die: Discover the Foods Scientifically Proven to Prevent and Reverse Disease.* New York: Flatiron, 2015. Print.

[11] Lipton, Bruce H. *The Honeymoon Effect: the Science of Creating Heaven on Earth.* Carlsbad, CA: Hay House, Inc., 2014.

[12] See, for example: Johnson, Caitlin. "Cutting Through Advertising Clutter." CBS News. CBS Interactive, September 17, 2006. https://www.cbsnews.com/news/cutting-through-advertising-clutter/

[13] Much of the information in this section originated from a discussion with my friend Anita Avalos, Certified Holistic Health, Eating Psychology, Body-Food Relationship Coach and yoga teacher.

[14] Anitaavalos.com

[15] Avena, Nicole M., Pedro Rada, and Bartley G. Hoebel. "Evidence for Sugar Addiction: Behavioral and Neurochemical Effects of Intermittent, Excessive Sugar Intake." *Neuroscience & Biobehavioral Reviews*32, no. 1 (2008): 20–39. https://doi.org/10.1016/j.neubiorev.2007.04.019.

[16] In *Guided by Your Own Stars* I discuss these topics at length.

[17] As usual, remember to consult your health care professional when considering doing a detox or making any major change, particularly if you are coming off of medications or are under care for an illness or entrenched health condition.

Chapter Three: What We Won't Be Eating

[18] Fitzgerald, Randall.*The Hundred-Year Lie: How to Protect Yourself from the Chemicals That Are Destroying Your Health.* New York: Plume, 2007.

[19] Ibid.

[20] Ibid.

[21] Ibid.

[22] Ibid.

[23] A great book to reference on this subject is: Siegel-Maier, Karyn. *The Naturally Clean Home.* North Adams, MA: Storey, 2009.

[24] "Organic Labeling." Organic Labeling | Agricultural Marketing Service. Accessed March 25, 2018. https://www.ams.usda.gov/rules-regulations/organic/labeling.

[25] Funk, Holly. "MaryJane Butters of MaryJanesFarm." Organic.org. July 15, 2005. Accessed March 25, 2018. http://www.organic.org/articles/showarticle/article-59.

[26] American Academy of Environmental Medicine (AAEM). Accessed February 26, 2020. https://www.aaemonline.org/gmo.php.

[27] "Labeling Around the World." Just Label It. Accessed March 26, 2018. http://www.justlabelit.org/right-to-know-center/labeling-around-the-world/.

[28] Allison Kopicki, "Strong Support for Labeling Modified Foods," *New York Times*, July 27, 2013. Foodandwaterwatch.org, a national watchdog organization, is a useful source of information like this.

[29] "BE Frequently Asked Questions - General." BE Frequently Asked Questions - General | Agricultural Marketing Service. Accessed March 13, 2020. https://www.ams.usda.gov/rules-regulations/be/faq/general.

[30] Just Label It. "Statement from Just Label It on USDA's Final Rule for Nationwide Disclosures of GMO Foods." Just Label It, December 20, 2018. http://www.justlabelit.org/press-room/statement-from-just-label-it-on-usdas-final-rule-for-nationwide-disclosures-of-gmo-foods/

[31] Market, Whole Foods. "Studies Show GMOs in Majority of U.S. Processed Foods, 58 Percent of Americans Unaware of Issue." PR Newswire: press release distribution, targeting, monitoring and marketing, June 30, 2018. https://www.prnewswire.com/news-releases/studies-show-gmos-in-majority-of-us-processed-foods-58-percent-of-americans-unaware-of-issue-104510549.html.

[32] Allen, Zuri. "Substantial Equivalence: The Who, What, When, Where, and Why." greenamerica.org, May 28, 2014. https://www.greenamerica.org/blog/substantial-equivalence-who-what-when-where-and-why

[33] Wilcks, Andrea, Bjarne Munk Hansen, Niels Bohse Hendriksen, and Tine Rask Licht. "Persistence of Bacillus Thuringiensis bioinsecticides in the Gut of Human-flora-associated Rats." *FEMS Immunology & Medical Microbiology*48, no. 3 (2006): 410-18. doi:10.1111/j.1574-695x.2006.00169.x.

[34] "Bt Corn: Health and the Environment - 0.707." Extension. Accessed March 26, 2018. http://extension.colostate.edu/topic-areas/agriculture/bt-corn-health-and-the-environment-0-707-2/.

[35] "Glyphosate Overview." GMO Free USA. Accessed March 26, 2018. https://gmofreeusa.org/research/glyphosate/glyphosate-overview/.

[36] "Glyphosate Studies." GMO Free USA. Accessed March 26, 2018.https://gmofreeusa.org/research/glyphosate/glyphosate-studies/.

[37] Glyphosate, Roundup, Glyphosate-Tolerance GM Soybeans, Chemical Extracted Soybean Food Oil/Soybean Powder Cause Serious Harm to

Health of American/Chinese People. Compiled and translated by I-wan, Chen (cheniwan@cei.gov.cn)

[38] For more information, MIT Professor Stephanie Seneff has compiled a list of resources and scientific articles located on her website https://people.csail.mit.edu/seneff/

[39] "Glyphosate Overview." GMO Free USA. Accessed March 26, 2018. https://gmofreeusa.org/research/glyphosate/glyphosate-overview/.

[40] "Union of Concerned Scientists Gives Monsanto an 'F' in Sustainable Agriculture." Union of Concerned Scientists, February 7, 2012. https://www.ucsusa.org/about/news/union-concerned-scientists-gives-monsanto-f-sustainable-agriculture

[41] Shiva, Vandana. *Stolen Harvest: The Hijacking of the Global Food Supply*. Cambridge, MA: South End, 2000. Print.

[42] For an extensive library of plant-based diet research, including over 700 articles, go to plantbasedresearch.org

[43] Gallagher, James. "Processed Meats Do Cause Cancer - WHO." BBC News. BBC, October 26, 2015. https://www.bbc.com/news/health-34615621.

[44] Greger, Michael, and Gene Stone. *How Not to Die: Discover the Foods Scientifically Proven to Prevent and Reverse Disease*. New York: Flatiron, 2015.

[45] Greger, Michael. "Uprooting the Leading Causes of Death." https://www.youtube.com/watch?v=30gEiweaAVQ&feature=youtu.be

[46] Campbell, T. Colin, and Thomas M. Campbell. *The China Study*. Dallas, TX: BenBella Books, 2005.

[47] Many mainstream documentaries, such as *Simply Raw, Forks Over Knives* and *Fat, Sick and Nearly Dead*, all document the benefits of a plant-based diet.

[48] Worldwatch Magazine, July/August 2004, Volume 17, No. 4

[49] Check out NOAA's website for current information on this massive problem: http://marinedebris.noaa.gov/info/patch.html

[50] "Vegetarianism and the Environment." Want to save the environment? Go vegetarian. Accessed February 26, 2020. http://michaelbluejay.com/veg/environment.html.

[51] Randall, Heather. "Exhausting the Planet: Jonathan Foley on Balancing Food Security With Environmental Sustainability." New Security Beat. Wilson Center, October 31, 2014. https://www.newsecuritybeat.org/2014/10/exhausting-planet-jon-foley-balancing-food-security-environmental-sustainability/.

[52] I cringe at the term "production" being used for live, sentient beings. Even the term "livestock" itself directly refers to ownership and an animal's use for human purposes, rather than referring to sentient, autonomous beings. In my opinion, our language could use an overhaul to reflect positive valuation and honoring of other species rather than enslavement and use-related labels—which is the topic of another book I've been working on.

[53] Tina. "Global Hunger: The More Meat We Eat, the Fewer People We Can Feed." Earthoria, March 25, 2008. http://www.earthoria.com/global-hunger-the-more-meat-we-eat-the-fewer-people-we-can-feed.html. Accessed February 26, 2020.

[54] Ibid.

Chapter Five: The Kitchen

[55] Environmental Working Group. "EWG's Tap Water Database: Contaminants in Your Water." EWG Tap Water Database | EWG Reviewed Contaminants. Accessed February 26, 2020. https://www.ewg.org/tapwater/ewg-reviewed-contaminants.php.

[56] https://www.chrisbeatcancer.com/wp-content/uploads/2011/05/other-juice-extractor-comparison-2007.pdf

[57] Although, after my second pregnancy I've found I can eat cashews again!

[58] "Natural" is defined by Whole Foods as "minimally processed foods that are free of hydrogenated fats as well as artificial flavors, colors, sweeteners, preservatives . . . " These foods also do not contain other "unacceptable food ingredients," a list of which can be found online. "Whole Foods Market." Wikipedia. Wikimedia Foundation, March 6, 2020. https://en.wikipedia.org/wiki/Whole_Foods_Market#cite_note-quality_standards-49.

[59] "Trader Joe's FAQs." Product Information | Trader Joe's. Accessed February 26, 2020. https://www.traderjoes.com/faqs/product-information.

[60] The Rawtarian recipes mobile app can be found at therawtarian.com

[61] Access at www.rawmazing.com

[62] Note: soy sauce is often used in Thai dishes and is usually not gluten free. If the place happens to have tamari on hand, this is also made from soy, but is not raw. Nama shoyu ("nama" means raw or unpasteurized) is *sometimes* raw. Sigh. This gets very tricky as some nama shoyu is heated above 115 degrees but is still claimed to contain living enzymes. For me, I eschew the analytics and just eat nama shoyu if I'm out and it's available. When at

home, I use coconut aminos, which have a similar (and to me, more pleasing) flavor, and are both raw and gluten free. I suppose I could carry these with me wherever I go, but, well, I just don't.

[63] See Chapter Nine: How to Travel and Dine in Raw Vegan Splendor for a thorough discussion.

[64] Clay, Rebecca A. "Green Is Good for You." Monitor on Psychology. American Psychological Association, April 2001. http://www.apa.org/monitor/apr01/greengood.aspx

[65] Ibid.

[66] The terms "superfood" and "superherb" refer to foods that are particularly nutrient dense and beneficial for health.

[67] For more information, I refer you to Vandana Shiva's work on soil entitled *Soil Not Oil*. Shiva, Vandana. *Soil Not Oil*. Berkeley, CA: North Atlantic Books, 2015.

[68] "Trans Fat: Double Trouble for Your Heart." Mayo Clinic. Mayo Foundation for Medical Education and Research, February 13, 2020. https://www.mayoclinic.org/diseases-conditions/high-blood-cholesterol/in-depth/trans-fat/art-20046114.

[69] Pollard, Kenneth Michael. "Silica, Silicosis, and Autoimmunity." *Frontiers in Immunology* 7 (November 2016). https://doi.org/10.3389/fimmu.2016.00097.

[70] Bell, Becky. "Food Dyes: Harmless or Harmful?". Healthline. January 7, 2017. https://www.healthline.com/nutrition/food-dyes

[71] Engeli, Roger, Simona Rohrer, Anna Vuorinen, Sonja Herdlinger, Teresa Kaserer, Susanne Leugger, Daniela Schuster, and Alex Odermatt. "Interference of Paraben Compounds with Estrogen Metabolism by Inhibition of 17β-Hydroxysteroid Dehydrogenases." *International Journal of Molecular Sciences* 18, no. 9 (2017): 2007. https://doi.org/10.3390/ijms18092007.

[72] Alban, Deane. "5 Neurotoxins Found in Popular Foods." Be Brain Fit. October 1, 2018. https://bebrainfit.com/neurotoxins-foods/

[73] "Talcum Powder and Cancer." American Cancer Society. Accessed February 26, 2020. https://www.cancer.org/cancer/cancer-causes/talcum-powder-and-cancer.html.

[74] Axe, Josh. "Most Supplements Contain Magnesium Stearate — Is It Safe?" Dr. Axe, September 4, 2019. https://draxe.com/nutrition/magnesium-stearate/.

[75] University of Zurich. "Titanium dioxide nanoparticles can exacerbate colitis." ScienceDaily. July 19, 2017.
www.sciencedaily.com/releases/2017/07/170719100521.htm

[76] https://www.framinghamheartstudy.org

[77] Campbell, T. Colin, and Thomas M. Campbell. *The China Study: The Most Comprehensive Study of Nutrition Ever Conducted and the Startling Implications for Diet, Weight Loss and Long-Term Health.* Dallas, TX: BenBella Books, 2017.

[78] https://www.forksoverknives.com/the-myth-of-complementary-protein/#gs.n4tO0Mc

[79] There are many oils on the market. However, Udo's Oil Blend is a particularly high quality product with a balance of the essential fatty acids or EFAs (EFAs are Omega 3 and Omega 6, which the body needs for survival but cannot synthesize and thus requires a direct source). Many EFA products contain fish oil, however, vegan versions such as Udo's Oil Blend can be found in most health food stores.

[80] See, for example:
"Raw Is Healing My Eyesight! - Health & Beauty Discussions on The Community Forum." The Community Forum.
https://www.therawtarian.com/community/f/discussion/5722/raw-is-healing-my-eyesight.

Index

About the Author

Christy Harden, M.S., M.A., is a certified Integrative Nutrition Coach through IIN and a Raw Food Consultant through raw food O.G. David Wolfe. She holds master's degrees in English and Speech Language Pathology, and a bachelor's in Environmental Studies. Christy is the author of the transformational how-to book *Guided by Your Own Stars* and the loving mother of two kiddos, her favorite "accomplishment" of all time. She works, plays and eats raw in Los Angeles.

You can connect with Christy at:

Website: www.christyharden.com
Facebook: www.facebook.com/ShaunChristy
Youtube.com: www.youtube.com/user/ShaunChristy

Also by Christy Harden

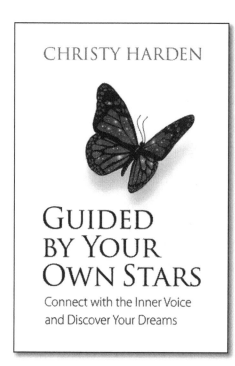

In order to live your dreams, you first need to know what they are.

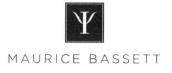

MAURICE BASSETT

Any number of books encourage you to "live the life of your dreams," but what if you don't know what those dreams are? *Guided by Your Own Stars* shows you, step by step, how to quiet the chaos and connect with your own intuitive knowing—the Inner Voice—to rediscover yourself and your dreams.

Use the blueprint in *Guided by Your Own Stars* to reconnect with your true essence and live a life of authenticity and joy.

This is your invitation to turn everything around, to get back to what matters to you, and to truly live your life.

Available in both paperback and audiobook
formats on Amazon.com

Publisher's Catalogue

The Prosperous Series

#1 The Prosperous Coach: Increase Income and Impact for You and Your Clients (Steve Chandler and Rich Litvin)

#2 The Prosperous Hip Hop Producer: My Beat-Making Journey from My Grandma's Patio to a Six-Figure Business (Curtiss King)

#3 The Prosperous Hotelier (David Lund)

* * *

Devon Bandison

Fatherhood Is Leadership: Your Playbook for Success, Self-Leadership, and a Richer Life

Roy G. Biv

Dancing on Rainbows: A Celebration of Numismatic Art

Sir Fairfax L. Cartwright

The Mystic Rose from the Garden of the King

Steve Chandler

37 Ways to BOOST Your Coaching Practice: PLUS: the 17 Lies That Hold Coaches Back and the Truth That Sets Them Free

50 Ways to Create Great Relationships

Business Coaching (Steve Chandler and Sam Beckford)

Crazy Good: A Book of CHOICES

CREATOR

Death Wish: The Path through Addiction to a Glorious Life

Fearless: Creating the Courage to Change the Things You Can

How to Get Clients (Revised Edition)

The Prosperous Coach: Increase Income and Impact for You and Your Clients (The Prosperous Series #1) (Steve Chandler and Rich Litvin)

RIGHT NOW: Mastering the Beauty of the Present Moment

Shift Your Mind Shift The World (Revised Edition)

Time Warrior: How to defeat procrastination, people-pleasing, self-doubt, over-commitment, broken promises and chaos

Wealth Warrior: The Personal Prosperity Revolution

Kazimierz Dąbrowski

Positive Disintegration

Charles Dickens

A Christmas Carol: A Special Full-Color, Fully-Illustrated Edition

Melissa Ford

Living Service: The Journey of a Prosperous Coach

James F. Gesualdi

Excellence Beyond Compliance: Enhancing Animal Welfare Through the Constructive Use of the Animal Welfare Act

Janice Goldman

Let's Talk About Money: The Girlfriends' Guide to Protecting Her ASSets

Sylvia Hall

This Is Real Life: Love Notes to Wake You Up

Christy Harden

Guided by Your Own Stars: Connect with the Inner Voice and Discover Your Dreams

I ♥ Raw: A How-To Guide for Reconnecting to Yourself and the Earth through Plant-Based Living

Curtiss King

The Prosperous Hip Hop Producer: My Beat-Making Journey from My Grandma's Patio to a Six-Figure Business (The Prosperous Series #2)

David Lindsay

A Blade for Sale: The Adventures of Monsieur de Mailly

David Lund

The Prosperous Hotelier (The Prosperous Series #3)

Abraham H. Maslow

The Aims of Education (audio)

The B-language Workshop (audio)

Being Abraham Maslow (DVD)

The Eupsychian Ethic (audio)

The Farther Reaches of Human Nature (audio)

Maslow and Self-Actualization (DVD)

Maslow on Management (audiobook)

Personality and Growth: A Humanistic Psychologist in the Classroom

Psychology and Religious Awareness (audio)

The Psychology of Science: A Reconnaissance

Self-Actualization (audio)

Weekend with Maslow (audio)

Harold E. Robles

Albert Schweitzer: An Adventurer for Humanity

Albert Schweitzer

Reverence for Life: The Words of Albert Schweitzer

William Tillier

Personality Development through Positive Disintegration: The Work of Kazimierz Dąbrowski

Margery Williams

The Velveteen Rabbit: or How Toys Become Real

Join our Mailing List:
www.MauriceBassett.com

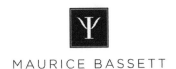

MAURICE BASSETT

Made in the USA
San Bernardino, CA
25 May 2020